How to Stay Fit as You Age

Kimberlee Bethany Bonura, Ph.D.

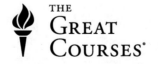

THE
GREAT
COURSES®

PUBLISHED BY:

THE GREAT COURSES
Corporate Headquarters
4840 Westfields Boulevard, Suite 500
Chantilly, Virginia 20151-2299
Phone: 1-800-832-2412
Fax: 703-378-3819
www.thegreatcourses.com

Kimberlee Bethany Bonura, Ph.D.

Fitness and Wellness Consultant

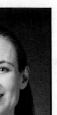

D
r. Kimberlee Bethany Bonura earned her Ph.D. in Educational Psychology from Florida State University, with a research focus in Sport and Exercise Psychology and graduate certificates in Program Evaluation and Educational Measurement and Statistics. Her doctoral dissertation, *The Impact of Yoga on Psychological Health in Older Adults*, won national awards from the American Psychological Association (Division 47) and the Association for Applied Sport Psychology (AASP).

Dr. Bonura serves as a peer reviewer and a member of the editorial board of the *International Journal of Yoga Therapy*. She is also a peer reviewer for the *Journal of Aging and Physical Activity*, *The Journal of Alternative and Complementary Medicine*, the *Journal of Asynchronous Learning Networks*, *The Journal of Social Change*, and the *Journal of Sport & Exercise Psychology*. Dr. Bonura serves as a member of the Master's Thesis Award Review Committee for the AASP and as a peer reviewer for the annual International Conference on College Teaching and Learning, as well as the annual conferences of the American Educational Research Association, the Canadian Psychological Association, and the American Psychological Association. She served as editor in chief of the Yoga Alliance newsletter *Yoga Matters* from 2002 to 2004.

Dr. Bonura has been practicing yoga since 1989 and teaching yoga since 1997. She is a triple-certified yoga instructor, registered with the Yoga Alliance, and a member of the International Association of Yoga Therapists. Dr. Bonura holds certifications as a personal trainer, group fitness instructor, kickboxing instructor, Tai Chi and Qigong instructor, senior fitness specialist, weight management instructor, and prenatal and youth fitness specialist. These certifications are issued by the Aerobics and Fitness Association of America and the International Fitness Professionals Association. She is also a Certified Anger Resolution Therapist and a Reiki Master in the Usui system.

Dr. Bonura has a line of instructional yoga and fitness DVDs that focus on older adult and adapted fitness programs. She has been published in local, national, and international magazines and journals in the topic areas of yoga, health, wellness, fitness, stress management, and performance enhancement. Dr. Bonura has developed specialized programs in seated/ chair yoga for senior citizens; pelvic yoga for pre- and postpregnancy, pre- and postmenopause, incontinence prevention, and sexual enhancement; yoga for empowerment, designed to encourage self-esteem in teenagers and young adults; and partner yoga for family and marital enhancement. She has consulted with individuals and organizations, including elite athletes, higher education institutions, nonprofit community organizations, and corporations. ■

Table of Contents

Table of Contents

Disclaimer

This series of lectures is intended to increase your knowledge of physiology, exercise, and health-related lifestyle choices and their basic effects on the human body as it ages. It is not designed for use as a medical reference to diagnose, treat, or prevent medical illnesses or trauma. Neither The Teaching Company nor Kimberlee Bethany Bonura is responsible for your use of this educational material or its consequences. If you have questions about the diagnosis, treatment, or prevention of a medical condition or illness, you should consult your personal physician.

How to Stay Fit as You Age

Scope:

Do you want to age, or do you want to age healthfully? A balanced fitness program will help you stay physically and psychologically healthy throughout your lifespan. You can cultivate a healthy body and a healthy mind through exercise. Whether you're already over 65, in your 50s but dealing with chronic conditions, or proactively planning ahead to stay healthy as you get older, the intent of this course is to support you in making good decisions that promote health and help you make the most of all the years you have. Whether you are just getting started with fitness or want to revitalize your existing fitness activities, this course will help you develop a plan to age healthfully.

To get the benefits of physical activity, you have to do it, and understanding motivational theory will help you leverage strategies for success. We will review barriers to change and stages-of-change theory to help you assess your current motivation level and establish a plan to get started.

Self-care is a vital part of health and wellness. Although self-care includes physical exercise, other considerations, such as stress management, a healthy diet, sufficient sleep, and mental exercise, all contribute to overall well-being. The consistent use of stress management techniques is an important part of any fitness program.

A balanced fitness program will help you stay physically and psychologically healthy throughout your lifespan. To support overall physical fitness, your exercise program should include cardiovascular exercise, strength and resistance training, flexibility training, balance training, and pelvic floor exercise. We will address the FITT principles (frequency, intensity, time, and type) to support you in developing the right plan for your current fitness level and your fitness goals.

You do not have to go to the gym to get fit. A broad array of activities supports physical fitness, including such activities of daily living as gardening and housekeeping. In fact, even if you exercise regularly, how much you sit will have an impact on your health. We will discuss workplace fitness and how you can better support your health in the office. We will also review opportunities to challenge yourself and expand your horizons through competitive sports and social fitness activities, such as dancing.

Mindfulness fitness practices are types of exercise intended to unify your mind and body through the combination of physical and psychological exercise. Mindful fitness practices include programs in yoga, Tai Chi, and the martial arts, all of which combine physical exercise with deliberate breathing and mental training. Mindful fitness practices provide physical fitness benefits, such as strength, flexibility, and balance training, but they also offer benefits beyond physical exercise. Research literature shows that mindfulness practices are particularly well suited to supporting mental health and well-being, helping to improve self-esteem, reducing depression and anxiety, and reducing perceptions of pain.

Our environments affect our fitness levels more than we may realize; the presence or absence of sidewalks and grocery stores, for instance, can influence the health-promoting decisions we make. If your environment does not set you up for success, then you are relying on willpower to push through in spite of obstacles. Research shows that we have limited reserves of willpower and that temptation and stress reduce our ability to exercise willpower; it's wise, then, to establish an environment that helps you conserve your willpower resources.

Having strong social relationships is also important for our health. In fact, in terms of risk for premature death, having a low level of social interaction is more harmful than not exercising, twice as harmful as being obese, and as harmful as smoking 15 cigarettes per day or being an alcoholic. When we have connections with other people, we have a greater sense of purpose, and that can help us feel motivated to take better care of ourselves and take fewer health risks.

When fitness and exercise become your central focus—when you live to exercise and eat healthfully—then you are no longer aging healthfully. If you find that the activities that should promote health are beginning to consume your life, you may have a problem. Even older adults are at risk for disordered behaviors, such as eating disorders, overtraining, and exercise addiction.

How you respond to illness, disability, or a chronic health condition will play a large part in determining your quality of life for the rest of your life. The times when exercise is hardest are when you just might need it the most. Adapted or modified physical fitness programs can help you recover more quickly and retain greater independence during illness, with chronic health conditions, and in spite of disabilities.

Physical activity promotes physical health. Benefits include improved energy and stamina; improved immune functioning and reduced risk for minor illnesses; and reduced risk for chronic conditions, such as diabetes, cardiovascular disease, and cancer. Physical activity also promotes psychological health; individuals who exercise regularly have a reduced risk for depression and anxiety and are more likely to experience marital satisfaction and earn higher pay. The goal of this course is to help you establish a plan for success that will enable you to reap these benefits, while having fun and maintaining your motivation.

This 12-lecture course is supported by 6 active sessions, including a relaxation session, a 30-minute chair yoga session; a 30-minute Tai Chi/Qigong session; a 30-minute foundational fitness session (including key strength and flexibility exercises); two 15-minute core strength and balance sessions (one chair based and one floor based); and three 10-minute workplace fitness sessions, one each for getting energized, managing stress, and simply standing up and moving. The relaxation session includes 15 minutes of progressive relaxation, 5 minutes of meditation using the anapana breathing technique, 5 minutes of meditation using alternate nostril breathing, and a 5-minute Reiki energy session. ■

Aging with Optimism—A Holistic Approach
Lecture 1

Aging happens. We are all getting older, and we must all face the physical realities that go with that fact. As we get older, we become more prone to illness, more susceptible to chronic conditions, and slower to heal and recover. There is no fountain of youth that will keep us as perpetually fit and healthy as most of us were at 18 or 25 or 30. But we can choose to stay active and to work through pain and illness. We can, in other words, take control of our aging and make deliberate decisions that will help us maintain independence, foster our well-being, promote health and happiness, and transform the experience of aging into healthy aging.

Defining "Old Age"

- According to the American College of Sports Medicine, the term "older adults" generally means individuals who are over age 65, but it can also be relevant for adults aged 50 to 64 who have "clinically significant chronic conditions or functional limitations that affect movement ability, fitness, or physical activity."

- For many of us, retirement and old age come sooner than we think they will. According to retirement survey statistics, only 23% of workers think they will retire before age 65, but 69% of retirees end up retiring before age 65. An earlier-than-planned retirement may be the result of a layoff, but it is often the result of unexpected health issues.

- Along with early retirement sometimes come unexpected limitations to our independence. For example, more than 20% of Americans over the age of 65 can no longer drive. On average, men live 7 years longer than they can drive, and women outlast their driving ability by 10 years.

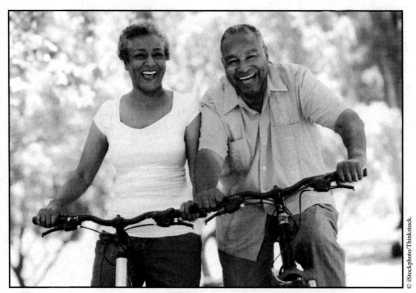

Happiness appears to be at its lowest between ages 51 and 55, after which it moves upward, with adults ages 66 to 70 reporting the highest levels of happiness.

- For all these reasons, it's important to think about how you're going to age, how you're going to deal with aging as it happens, and what you can do to age as healthfully as possible.

The Aging Process

- Even in the absence of disease, structural and functional deterioration occur in most physiological systems. These age-related changes affect a broad range of tissues, organ systems, and functions, and together, these changes affect activities of daily living and physical independence.

- Physiological aging includes declines in maximal aerobic capacity and skeletal muscle performance; thus, a fit man of 25 will run faster than a fit man of 65. But across the range of capacity, we determine where we are with our own levels of activity and exercise.
  - Although a 22-year-old man in peak physical condition has higher aerobic and muscle capacity than a 66-year-old man in

peak physical condition, the 66-year-old man is more capable and fit than a 22-year-old man who doesn't exercise or take care of himself.

○ In fact, where you are on the spectrum of capacity now can predict where you will be later. Baseline values of physical fitness in middle-aged adults can predict future risks of disability, chronic disease, and death.

• Physiological aging also includes changes in body composition. Between the ages of 18 and 55, the average sedentary American gains between 17 and 20 pounds of fat. Between 55 and 65, we gain another 2 to 5 pounds of fat.

○ This gradual accumulation of body fat is accompanied by a redistribution of fat to central (around the middle) and visceral (internal) locations during middle age. We also experience a loss of muscle, called sarcopenia, during middle and older age.

○ These changes cause a domino effect: As you gain fat weight and lose muscle mass, your metabolism slows, causing you to gain more weight.

• Age-related changes in hormones affect how we store fat and burn calories and how much muscle mass we have. For instance, before menopause, women are more likely to store fat around the hips and thighs. After menopause, changes in estrogen levels make women more likely to store fat around the middle, which puts them at greater risk for cardiovascular disease.

○ But this cascade is not inevitable. Changes in diet and exercise can affect how much weight you gain and store. Resistance exercise can help you maintain or rebuild muscle mass.

○ Exercise to burn fat and build muscle improves your resting metabolic rate, helping you to burn more calories even while at rest.

- Getting older appears to be associated with declining levels of physical activity. The American College of Sports Medicine reports that older adults are generally less physically active than younger adults. Further, active older adults may spend almost as much time in physical activity as active younger adults, but they participate in lower-intensity activities, such as walking, gardening, and golf.

- Another normal consequence of aging is increased risk for illness and chronic disease. Advanced age is a risk factor for cardiovascular disease, type II diabetes, obesity, certain cancers, osteoporosis, and arthritis. All other things being equal, older adults are more likely to deal with these issues. But regular physical activity substantially modifies your risk profile for all these conditions.

    o Compared to their peers, older athletes demonstrate many physiological and health advantages. They have a more favorable body composition profile, with less total body fat and less abdominal fat; greater muscle mass; and higher bone mineral density. They are also 30% to 50% stronger than their sedentary peers and have improved aerobic fitness.

    o Older athletes have a reduced coronary risk profile, including lower blood pressure, better insulin sensitivity, lower levels of inflammation, and healthier levels of fats in the blood, all of which make them less susceptible to cardiovascular disease, heart attack, and stroke. Further, older adult athletes have faster nerve conduction velocity, meaning that they maintain better reaction time, which can have implications for holding on longer to their car keys.

    o Older adults who are active also are slower to develop disability in old age, meaning that even though aging occurs in athletic adults, it happens at a slower pace and is less likely to lead to the same levels of dependence and loss of ability.

Locus of Control

- Locus of control is the extent to which a person believes that he or she can influence the environment. Research has demonstrated that people with an internal locus of control are healthier and more successful in adhering to health programs. People with an external locus of control may feel powerless and are at greater risk for illness.

- It is our internal perspective that matters because our happiness levels have a way of adapting to our circumstances. For instance, research with lottery winners shows that a few months after the excitement wears off, people are back to the happiness levels they had before they won. The same holds true for people who have experienced trauma, such as the loss of a limb or the death of a spouse; within a few years, they return to the same happiness levels they had before the traumatic event.

- Likewise, our mindset may determine how old we feel. In one study done in the early 1980s, older men were taken to a retreat that was set up to reflect the 1950s. One group of men was instructed to talk and interact as if they were living in the 1950s, while the other group was instructed to reminisce about their youth. Both groups improved in physical and mental tests from being reconnected to their youthful selves, but the group that lived as if they were young again improved even more. Living younger prompted their bodies to act younger!

No Pain, No Gain or No Pain, No Pain?

- In starting an exercise program, it's important to seek a balanced approach. Take the long view and move forward slowly.

- For some people, a degree of pain may be inevitable. If you live with chronic pain, you have to work through the discomfort of exercise—even accept it—so that you can use that discomfort to create health benefits that may reduce your pain in the long run. You must learn to be comfortable with discomfort as part of the growth process.

- Of course, you'll notice that these are two opposing views: On the one hand, you don't want to exercise to the point of pain or injury.

Bellows Breath

The Stomach Pump or "Bellows Breath" is a yoga exercise you can do anywhere. This exercise focuses on active engagement of the abdominal muscles, strengthening your core and promoting a healthier digestive system.

Start by assuming a comfortable position with good posture. Ideally, you're standing, but you can also remain seated. Your feet should be wide and balanced, chest open, and shoulders rolled down and back.

Bend forward gently from the waist, place your hands on your knees, and take a deep inhalation. Then, exhale completely, pulling your belly button back to your spine.

Once you've exhaled, pause, without breath, and actively contract your stomach in and out, like a fireplace bellows. Relax, inhale, exhale out completely, and contract your stomach again.

On the other hand, if you live with chronic pain, you have to work through the discomfort you will feel while exercising to improve your health.

Fitness Goals
- For older adults, the goals of a fitness program can be confusing. Are you exercising to recapture abilities you used to have or to maintain what you've got? The answer may depend on your health and current fitness levels.
  - If you have not been deliberate about health and exercise in your youth, you may find that through a deliberate focus on fitness, you will experience better health in your older years than you did when you were younger.

  - In contrast, for older people who have always been fit, some of the inevitable physical changes of aging can be particularly difficult. As you age, you need to accept that fitness looks different.

- When centenarians are studied, researchers find that their longevity is generally due to a healthy lifestyle. Above all, three specific health-promoting characteristics stand out: (1) They exercise regularly; (2) they maintain a positive mental attitude; and (3) they maintain a good social network. We'll focus on these three components throughout this course.

- For many of us, one of the hardest things about getting older is a loss of perceived control. But perceptions of control over your own life are directly related to psychological health and well-being.
  - Because of this, exercise scientists believe that many of the benefits of exercise for older adults may be related to the degree to which exercise helps us maintain a sense of psychosocial control, self-efficacy, and perceived competency.

  - In turn, these attitudes can predict how well we will sustain behavior changes. In other words, if we feel as if we can get healthy, we are more likely to stick to the behaviors that make us healthy.

- As we go through this course together, remember that you can have an impact on your health and well-being. You can make the choice to be active and fit. You can stay engaged in your life until your very last breath. You may or may not be able to change your health, your finances, or your life circumstances, but you can choose to make the most and the best of what you've got in order to experience healthy aging.

Suggested Reading

Cozolino, *The Healthy Aging Brain*.

Langer, *Counterclockwise*.

Weil, *Healthy Aging*.

Activities and Assignments

Consider going to your doctor for a physical and to discuss your health status and safety precautions for exercise.

Dedicate a journal or notebook for your activities with this course.

Complete a personal inventory. Assess:
- Your current health status

- Your fears and preconceived notions about your health status

- Your current activity level

- Your obstacles to health and fitness

- What health aging means to you.

Aging with Optimism—A Holistic Approach
Lecture 1—Transcript

Imagine two women, both in their late 70s. The first woman lives an active life. She and her husband live with her adult daughter's family, and are actively involved in caring for their grandchild and the family's two dogs. Every day, she goes for a two-mile walk with her daughter. She cleans the house, cooks dinner every night, and bakes bread from scratch every week. She gardens, she travels around the world with her daughter's family, and volunteers in her granddaughter's school and in the community senior citizen program. For fun, she paints with oils and acrylics; she knits, crochets, and sews.

The second woman is plagued by both chronic and acute illness. After stomach and uterine cancer in her 50s, she had a hysterectomy and partial removal of her stomach. Chronic rheumatoid arthritis, severe osteoporosis, and degeneration of her spine mean she lives with chronic pain. She has type-2 diabetes and glaucoma, and she's had to have cataract surgery in both eyes. She has high blood pressure and high cholesterol, and has survived a couple of strokes and a heart attack.

Is the second woman just unlucky? Does she have bad genes? Is she suffering from bad choices?

Would you believe me if I told you that they were the same woman? I'm talking about my grandmother, and she had really poor health. And her poor health was the result of a combination of bad luck, bad genes, and bad choices. But in spite of it, she chose to live an active, engaged life, and make the most of the time she had. She lived until she was 85, and I was lucky to have her to set a good example.

When my grandfather passed away 15 months before my grandmother did, to stay active and find something positive to focus on, she, my mom, and I all took ballroom dance lessons together. About 10 months before she died, we had one last three-generations adventure. We took her to Paris to see the Louvre; we went to the beaches in the south of France. And then, with a little help from hospice in her last few months, we were able to care for her at home until she passed away.

Aging happens. We are all getting older and there are some physical realities that go with that. Let me give you a personal example. I've been teaching yoga since I was 19, and in my early 20s, I taught 15–20 yoga classes a week, and did another 10–15 hours of yoga in my own practice each week. Needless to say, I was both very strong and very flexible. I would go to advanced yoga classes with other teachers, and I could pop into any yoga pose they taught. Without even warming up, I could go into a backbend so deep that I brought my toes to my forehead.

Other students called me Gumby, and one teacher liked to use me as a human doll and move my limbs into advanced stretches. I knew that my flexibility was the result of all the yoga I did, but I also thought it came naturally, and I didn't realize how much life, injury, and aging would affect it. In my 30s, I've spent significant chunks of time where it was medically contraindicated for me to do abdominal exercises or backbends. And so now—even though I still do yoga regularly, most of the time every day, and at least several days per week—and even though I have a lot of strength and flexibility, no one would mistake me for Gumby anymore. Every bit of strength and flexibility I have, I am fully aware of how hard I have had to work to rebuild it, and then continue working to keep it.

As we get older, we become more prone to illness, more susceptible to chronic conditions, slower to heal and recover. There is no fountain of youth that will keep us as perpetually fit and healthy as most of us were at 18 or 25 or 30. We will frame our discussion for his course in that realism because within that frame of realism, we have so many wonderful choices about the picture we can paint.

We can choose to stay active. We can choose to make good decisions that will keep us engaged—engaged with life and the people we love. We can choose to give into pain and illness, or we can work through them and discover that we have more strength than we thought, different abilities than we previously knew we had. We have more opportunity for wisdom, for kindness, for self-awareness. We can be more and better because we are older. In fact, because we are older, we're even more likely to be happy. Research has found that older adults have the highest levels of happiness. Happiness appears to be at its lowest between ages 51 and 55 and then it moves upward, with adults aged 66–70 reporting the highest levels of happiness. How happy you feel may also be directly tied to how healthy you are—people who indicate they are in good or excellent health are three times more likely than others to report being very happy. So, we can just give in and age—it's going to happen anyway—or we can take control of our aging, and make deliberate decisions that will help us to maintain our independence, foster our well-being, promote our health and happiness, and transform our experience of aging into healthy aging.

What do we mean, then, when we say "old age"? According to the American College of Sports Medicine Position Stand on Exercise and Physical Activity for Older Adults, the term "older adults" generally means individuals over age 65, but can also be relevant for adults aged 50–64 who have "clinically significant chronic conditions or functional limitations that affect movement ability, fitness, or physical activity."

For many of us, retirement and old age come sooner than we think. According to retirement survey statistics, only 23 percent of workers think they will retire before age 65, but 69 percent of retirees end up retiring before age 65. An earlier-than-planned retirement may be the result of a layoff, but it is often due to unexpected health issues. And with that early retirement sometimes comes limitations to our independence that we aren't expecting: More than 20 percent of Americans over the age of 65 can no longer drive. One older adult advocacy group anticipates that by 2015 more than 15 ½ million adults over the age of 65 will live in areas with no public transportation. On average, men live seven years longer than they can drive; women outlast their driving ability by ten years. So it's important to think about how we're going to age, how we're going to deal with aging as it happens, and what we can do to age as healthfully as possible.

Whether you're already over 65, in your 50s but dealing with chronic conditions, or proactively planning ahead to stay healthy as you get older, the intent of this course is to support you in making good decisions that promote health and help you make the most of all the years you have.

Let's talk a little about the aging process. Even in the absence of disease, structural and functional deterioration occurs in most physiological systems. These age-related changes affect a broad range of tissues, organ systems, and functions, and together, these changes affect activities of daily living and physical independence. So in layman's terms, no matter what, we're all getting older. And even if we stay healthy, there are normal changes that happen as part of the aging process.

Let's review some of these changes that happen with aging, so that we can talk about aging and how we can use fitness activities to support the highest level of functioning and independence possible, across your lifespan. We will talk about activities and strategies in this course that you can use to turn aging into healthy aging.

Physiological aging includes declines in maximal aerobic capacity and skeletal muscle performance. What that means is that a fit man of 25 will run faster than a fit man of 65. But—across the range of capacity—we determine where we are, with our own levels of activity and exercise. That 22-year-old man in peak physical condition has a higher aerobic capacity and muscle capacity than a 66-year-old man in peak physical condition, but the 66-year-old man in peak physical condition is more capable and fit than a 22-year-old who doesn't exercise and doesn't take care of himself.

In fact, where we are on the spectrum of our capacity now can predict where we will be later: Baseline values of physical fitness in middle-aged adults can actual predict future risks of disability, chronic disease, and death. How well you care for yourself now has a long-term impact.

Another aspect of physiological aging is changes in body composition. Between the ages of 18 and 55 years, the average sedentary American will gain between 17 and 20 pounds of fat. Between 55 and 65, we will gain another 2 to 5 pounds of fat. So there is this gradual accumulation of body fat, and a redistribution of fat to central (around your middle) and visceral (internal) locations during middle age. There is also a loss of muscle, called sarcopenia, during middle and older age. And then it's a domino effect—as you gain fat weight and lose muscle mass, your metabolism slows, which causes you to gain more weight.

Age-related changes in hormones affect how we store fat and burn calories, and how much muscle mass we have. For instance, before menopause, women are more likely to store fat around the hips and thighs. After menopause, changes in estrogen make women more likely to store fat around the middle. You go from a pear to an apple. Being an apple tends to put you at greater risk for cardiovascular disease.

But this cascade is not inevitable. Changes in diet and exercise can affect how much weight you gain and store. Resistance exercise can help you maintain or rebuild muscle mass. You can use exercise to burn fat and build muscle, which will then improve your resting metabolic rate, helping you to burn more calories even while at rest.

It's never too late to get active. Research shows that improvements in aerobic capacity occur after aerobic exercise training even in adults over age 75. One small study with frail, institutionalized adults over the age of 90 found that just 8 weeks of resistance training led to strength gains of 174 percent, and increased their walking speeds by 48 percent. If frail adults over 90 years old living in a nursing home can get stronger through exercise, then we can all do it! We'll talk more about the basic components you should include in your fitness program in Lecture 4. Our active session on foundational fitness includes resistance exercises that you can use to maintain or rebuild your strength.

Getting older appears to be associated with declining levels of physical activity. The American College of Sports Medicine reports that older adults are generally less physically active than younger adults are. Active older adults may spend almost as much time in physical activity as active younger adults, but they participate in lower-intensity activities like walking, gardening, and golf. However, I'm not convinced that we become less active because we're getting older. Rather, I think that part of why we lose ability and health as we get older is because we're becoming less active. In Lecture 5, we'll talk about the physical health benefits of daily activity, and how important they are in your overall fitness and wellness plan. You can also try a few forms of exercise that you've likely heard a lot about—we've included a Chair Yoga and a Qigong session in our active lectures.

Another normal consequence of aging is an increased risk for illness and chronic disease. Advanced age is a risk factor for cardiovascular disease, type-2 diabetes, obesity, certain cancers, osteoporosis, and arthritis. All other things being equal, older adults are more likely to deal with these issues. But regular physical activity substantially modifies your risk profile for all of these conditions. In fact, the American College of Sports Medicine proposes that the primary reason exercise increases life expectancy is because of its positive influence on the development of chronic disease.

One way to understand the extensive benefits of exercise is to compare older adult athletes with age-matched peers. Compared to their peers, older adult athletes demonstrate many physiological and health benefits. They have a more favorable body composition profile, with less total body fat and less abdominal fat. They have greater muscle mass, and higher bone mineral density. They are also 30–50 percent stronger than their sedentary peers are. They have improved aerobic fitness, including more oxidative and fatigue-resistant limb muscles, a higher capacity to transport and use oxygen, a higher cardiac stroke volume at peak exertion, and a younger pattern of left ventricular filling—all of which means that they are more able to do aerobic exercise like walking, biking, and swimming for longer, and with less fatigue.

They also have a reduced coronary risk profile: lower blood pressure, better insulin sensitivity, lower levels of inflammation, healthier levels of fats in the blood, with lower triglycerides, lower low-density lipoprotein cholesterol and total cholesterol, and higher high-density lipoprotein cholesterol—all of which make them less susceptible to cardiovascular disease, heart attack, and stroke. Further, older adult athletes have faster nerve conduction velocity—meaning that they maintain better reaction time and reactivity. That can have implications for when you have to give up your car keys. Older adults who are active also are slower to develop disability in old age—meaning that while aging still happens, even to athletic adults, it happens at a slower pace, and is less likely to lead to the same levels of dependence or loss of ability.

In Lecture 11, we'll talk more about the physical and the psychological benefits of exercise, and discuss how regular exercise can reduce your risk for both chronic and acute illness. The nice part about looking at how exercise can promote health and fitness is that a little goes a long way. As the Centers for Disease Control and Prevention slogan goes: "10 minutes at a time is fine!" Shoot for a minimum of 150 minutes of exercise per week, and you can break it up into manageable 10-minute chunks. Three 10-minute blocks of physical activity each day, at least 5 days per week, are sufficient to provide health benefits. Just 30 minutes, five days a week in three 10-minute blocks. Sure, more is better—and more will get you even more health benefits. And if you really want to lose weight or get really fit, you have to do more. But do something. Get started!

We have active lectures in this course to provide you with some supportive opportunities to get started and try different types of fitness. They are sequenced in a supportive structure—first we focus on relaxation strategies, to help you manage your stress. Then, you have the opportunity to learn more about the fundamental components of fitness, particularly stretching and resistance training. We also include two core body workouts—one on a chair for those with mobility limitations, and one on the floor for a more challenging workout. There are also three brief 10-minute workouts that you can fit into your day, even at work, so that you can make those three 10-minute blocks of exercise easy to achieve. Finally, there are two full 30-minute workouts, one for Chair Yoga and one for Qigong, so that you can try these mindful fitness practices for yourself to experience their benefits.

Let's try something small and simple right now, so that you can see how even a few moments of exercise can help you to feel better. As we get older, we notice a lot of differences around our midsection. Our digestive system gets fussier—we can't eat the junk and the spicy food as easily or drink as much without suffering the consequences. We have to be grownups and take fiber to promote regularity and reduce our cholesterol. Our belts get a little tighter, even if we're careful with diet and exercise.

There is a wonderful yoga exercise called the Stomach Pump or the Bellows Breath, which focuses on the active engagement of your abdominal muscles. You can do anywhere—no gym clothes or special equipment required.

Start by coming into a comfortable position with good posture. Ideally, you're standing, but if you want to stay seated, that's fine too. Your feet are wide and balanced, your chest is open, shoulders rolled down and back. Bend forward gently from the waist and place your hands on your knees. Take a nice deep inhalation.

Now, exhale completely, pulling your belly button back to your spine. Once your breath is out—pause there, without breath, and then actively contract your stomach in and out, like a fireplace bellows. Now relax—inhale again. Exhale out completely, belly button back to the spine, and pump your stomach. Let's do one more—inhale—exhale, belly button to the spine, and pump.

I've had yoga students say that this one exercise made a difference in their waistline, and in their whole experience of their digestive system. If you're feeling sluggish or constipated, try doing five of these each morning and five each evening, and pay attention to how your internal body seems to move better. We'll talk more about core body fitness, and exercises that you can do to strengthen your core, in the core active sessions.

What we're doing is starting with the idea of fitness for health promotion. When you're feeling stronger, better, and more motivated, then we can start thinking about fitness for fitness promotion. Throughout this course, we'll talk about the skills and strategies you can use both to get started with fitness, and to sustain your fitness program throughout your lifespan.

Research has demonstrated that people with an internal locus of control are healthier and more successful in adhering to health programs. Locus of control is the extent to which a person believes he or she can influence the environment. People with an external locus of control may feel powerless and are at a greater risk for illness.

It really is our internal perspective that matters, because our happiness levels have a way of adapting to our circumstances. For instance, research with lottery winners has found that a few months after the excitement wears off, people are back to the happiness level they had before they won. The same holds true with negative circumstances. Research shows that even the effects of something as traumatic as the loss of a limb or the death of a spouse are short-lived—within a few years, you're back to the same happiness level you had before the traumatic event. So there are miserable millionaires, and contented amputees, precisely because most of what really matters is what's in our own heads.

My mother has a friend named Anna who is a sweet, kind lady, just barely making it on Social Security. But she loves her extended family of children and grandchildren and great-grandchildren and is always happy and welcoming. Years ago, my mom was dating a man who was quite well off—he owned a bar and a restaurant in the New York City area—and she brought him with her to a family party at Anna's house. When they left, he was visibly angry, and he said, "She has nothing, and lives in this rundown apartment—but she's happier than me. That's not fair!" So for all his physical riches, she was the one who is truly rich because she has happiness that she's built with the people she loves.

Likewise, our mindset may actually determine how old we feel. In one fascinating study done in the early 1980s by Harvard psychologist Ellen Langer, older men were taken to a retreat that was set up to reflect the 1950s. The magazines, newspapers, TV, radio, and music were all from the 1950s, and there were no indications of the present time. One group of men was instructed to talk and interact as if it was the 1950s, and to talk about everything in the present tense. The other group was instructed to reminisce about their youth in the 50s. Both groups took physical and mental tests of grip strength, manual dexterity, posture, gait, memory, hearing and vision both before and after the retreat. And both groups improved across all measures, from being reconnected to their youthful selves—but the group that lived as if it was the 1950s, as if they were young again, improved even more. By living younger, their bodies actually acted as if they were younger! Some of the men even put down their canes by the end of the week and started playing touch football! So how we think about aging—and how we think about ourselves in the aging process—can have a profound impact on how we will age.

We'll spend a lot of time throughout our lectures talking about our emotions, our relationships, and our motivations. What's in our heads and our hearts has a profound impact on our fitness and our wellness. Motivation is the foundation for everything we do—because it doesn't matter how much exercise can help your health, if you're not motivated to exercise. In Lectures 2, 7, and 12, we'll focus on how you can build, support, and sustain your motivation for fitness.

Years ago in El Paso, I had a great Qigong instructor, who said that he never liked the American ideal of "no pain, no gain." He preferred to live by "no pain, no pain!" That's such a nice, true way to philosophize about exercise, because exercise to the point of pain puts you at risk for injury—it makes you likely to over train, to overdo—and then, because you're injured, you'll actually do less. So what I would like to do is encourage you to seek a balanced approach. To take the long view and move forward slowly. Let's be tortoises, not hares. We'll talk more about overtraining, and how to stay safe while you exercise, in Lecture 9.

There are some times, though, when pain is inevitable—for instance, the pain of chronic conditions. If you're living with chronic pain, you have to work through the discomfort of exercise—even accept it—so that you can use that discomfort to create health benefits that may actually reduce your pain in the long run. You have to be comfortable with discomfort as part of the growth process.

So really, I'm talking about two opposing views, both intended to get you to good health. On the one hand, you don't want to exercise to the point of pain. You don't want to injure yourself and make it impossible for you to exercise. On the other hand, if you live with chronic pain, you have to work through that discomfort that you will feel while exercising in order to actually improve your health. It can seem unfair, I know—if you're healthy I'm telling you that exercise won't hurt and shouldn't hurt. If you're in chronic pain, I'm telling you to add one more uncomfortable task to your life. But we'll talk more in Lecture 10, about how to use exercise based on your condition, so that you experience the least discomfort possible, and we'll talk about how exercise to actually improve your condition and reduce your pain in the long run. As well, we offer a Chair Yoga session in our active lectures, which is adapted to be accessible to everyone, even those with limited mobility.

As we get older, there is confusion about what the goals of a fitness program should be. Is it to recapture abilities we used to have? To maintain what we've got? That may depend on your health and your current fitness levels. If you have not been deliberate about health and exercise in your youth, you may actually find that through a deliberate focus on fitness, you will experience better health in your older years than you did when you were young.

Some of the inevitable physical changes can be particularly difficult for older people who have always been fit. It can be difficult to accept that as you age, fitness is going to look different.When centenarians—people who live to be over 100 years old—are studied, researchers find that their longevity is generally due to a healthy lifestyle. And above all, three specific health-promoting characteristics stand out. First, they exercise regularly. Second, they maintain a positive mental attitude. Third, they maintain a good social network.

Throughout this course, we'll focus a great deal on all three components. The primary focus is how to use exercise to stay fit as we age, but our mental health—that positive attitude of centenarians—and our social health and connections with others also influence our fitness. We'll talk more about both, to support you in developing a holistic view of healthy aging. We'll also talk about self-care in general, and how you can support a holistic view of aging through stress management and other good decisions like getting enough sleep. We also offer several relaxation and stress-management activities in the active lectures, to support your overall health and well-being.

For many of us, one of the hardest things about getting older is a loss of perceived control. Independence that we fought to gain when we were young, we fight to hold onto as we get old. Perceptions of control over your own life are directly related to both psychological health and well-being. Because of this, exercise scientists believe that many of the benefits of exercise as we get older may be related to how exercise helps us maintain a sense of psychosocial control, self-efficacy, and perceived competency. This sense of improved control, self-efficacy, and competency can actually predict how well we will sustain behavior changes. In other words, if we feel like we can get healthy, we are more likely to stick to the behaviors that make us healthy.

If you remember nothing else from this course, I hope you will remember that you can have an impact on your health and well-being. You can make the choice to be active and be fit. You can stay engaged in your life until your very last breath. You may or may not be able to change your health, your finances, or your life circumstances. But you can choose to make the most and the best of what you've got, in order to experience healthy aging.

We will work together so that you can set a plan to experience the benefits of healthy aging. I encourage you to use this program to meet your needs, and to help you accomplish your personal aging agenda. Before we get started, you may want to see your doctor and get a physical. To plan the fitness program that is right for you, you need to start with a baseline understanding of your health, and any health concerns that may impact how you exercise. Consider talking to your doctor about your intent to begin an exercise program, and follow any advice or guidance he or she offers to keep you safe as you get fit.

Throughout this course, we will do concrete exercises to help you personalize the strategies so that you can successfully implement them in your life. You may want to get a new notebook or journal that you dedicate just to this program. We'll use it throughout the lectures, with activities designed to put theory into practice. In our final lecture, we'll also talk about how you can continue to use your journal to support your ongoing commitment to healthy aging.

The first activity I'd like you to do is to start with an inventory. Take some time, and really reflect on each of the following. Get yourself off to a good start by being really reflective, and really honest with yourself. Take at least 15 to 30 minutes per question, so that you have a good sense of where you are, and where you want to go.

Think about the following: What is your current health status? What acute illnesses or conditions are you currently dealing with? What chronic illnesses or conditions do you have? What strategies have you already tried?

Then ask yourself: What are your fears and preconceived notions about your health status? What do you believe you can or can't achieve, based on the examples others have set for you? How did your parents age. What impact did that have on your perception of aging?

Consider: What's your current activity level? How much physical activity do you already do each day, each week, each month? How much physical exercise do you deliberately do each day, each week, each month?]

Also consider: What are your obstacles to health and fitness? What is preventing you from leading the active life you wish you could lead? Think about internal factors, such as your health or your beliefs, and external factors like your environment or your circumstances.

And then, most importantly of all, reflect on: What does healthy aging mean to you? What does your ideal life look like, in terms of your health, your fitness, and your activity? Be both realistic and optimistic, and identify the goals you want to achieve now, over the next year, and over the next decade.

I want to make one more thing really clear, to set us off on the right foot on this path together. I can provide information and resources. I will be your guide, your support, and your mentor on this journey—but you must do the work. You must put it into practice. You must make the choice to experience healthy aging. If you're with me, then let's start our journey together.

Getting and Staying Motivated
Lecture 2

Although most of us know the benefits of physical activity, few of us are sufficiently active. In fact, research shows that more than 80% of adults do not meet minimal guidelines for recommended physical activity and as many as 34% of older adults are completely inactive. What is it that gets us moving? A fundamental component is motivation—the desire and will to do something. In this lecture, we'll discuss a model of behavior change, the many obstacles to change we all face, and the kinds of personal motivators that can get you moving.

Transtheoretical Model of Behavior Change

- The transtheoretical model of behavior change, or stages-of-change theory, holds that when faced with a potential change, our motivation falls into one of six stages: (1) precontemplation, (2) contemplation, (3) preparation, (4) action, (5) maintenance, and (6) termination. Let's walk through each of these stages, using a smoker as an example to illustrate each stage.

- In the precontemplation stage, a person is not ready for change and may not even be aware that his or her behavior is problematic. A smoker in precontemplation has no intention of quitting smoking.

- An individual in the contemplation stage is getting ready for change. This is someone who is starting to recognize that he or she may have a problem. The individual

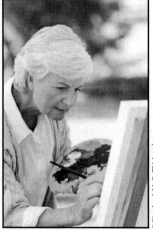

Research shows that our capacity for imagination can help us make better decisions, including decisions about healthy aging.

expends cognitive energy looking at the pros and cons of the behavior to determine whether to make a change. Perhaps the smoker has a new grandchild, and the grandchild's pediatrician has provided information about the dangers of third-hand smoke. The grandparent may begin to think of smoking as more troublesome than it seemed earlier.

- An individual in the preparation stage intends to take action in the immediate future and may even begin to take small steps toward change. The smoker may make an appointment at a smoking cessation clinic or buy a box of nicotine gum or patches. These are preparatory steps toward making a change.

- When the individual actually begins to make the change, through specific, overt behavior modifications, he or she has moved into the action phase. Our smoker is wearing the patch or chewing nicotine gum and hasn't smoked a cigarette in several days. The smoker may also make adjustments in his or her life to better support the change, such as having the carpets cleaned or practicing self-hypnosis or meditation to work through stress instead of smoking.

- After several successful months as a nonsmoker, the former smoker moves into the maintenance phase. The individual has maintained the new, healthy behavior for a substantive period of time but is still actively working to prevent a relapse.

- At some point, maintenance moves to termination—the stage in which the individual is no longer tempted to relapse. Some psychologists believe that termination occurs when a behavior has been successfully maintained for at least 1 year.

- It's important to note, however, that for some behaviors, such as addiction to drugs, alcohol, or smoking, relapse can occur even after years of maintenance. Because of this, some psychologists believe that a changed individual is always in maintenance and will always have to actively work to maintain the healthy behavior.

Barriers to Change

- The topic of motivation also encompasses the obstacles—barriers to change—that get in the way of doing what we set out to do.

- One common barrier to change is procrastination, which in many cases, may be connected to a fear of perfection. We worry that we aren't good enough or that we can't do something well enough, so we give up before we even try. But generally in life—and certainly when we are talking about our health—good enough really is good enough. It's better to accept good enough than to keep waiting for perfection.

- Instant gratification is another barrier to change. You may want to make healthy choices, but it's more fun to watch TV, have a snack, read a book, or take a nap. Remember, though, that "easy" is not the same thing as "gratifying." It may take a little push to get you out the door for a walk, but once you're walking, you will actually feel good from the fresh air, the activity, and the sunshine.

- Preconditioned beliefs can also be barriers to change. Perhaps you believe that you're not an athlete, that exercise is undignified for older adults, or that you might get hurt if you exercise. The key here is to question these beliefs. Who says you're not an athlete? Why can't you be both dignified and fit? If you worried that you might get hurt, make fitness choices that are gentle and have a low potential for risk.

- Still another common belief is that a little exercise won't make a difference, but the truth is that it does. A large study published in 2008 in the *British Journal of Sports Medicine* reported that just 20 minutes of physical activity per week is sufficient to promote mental health. And taking a moderate 30-minute walk 5 times a week is enough exercise to significantly reduce your risk of dying prematurely.

- Fear of discomfort is also a common barrier to change, and it's true that exercise can be uncomfortable and make you tired. But if you choose an exercise program that is right for your body, abilities, and interests, you'll find that being uncomfortable isn't the same as being pain. You'll also learn that some discomfort—some sense of muscle fatigue—is normal and is part of the process of becoming stronger and have less chronic pain.

- For some people, globalizing is a barrier to change. Those who have had one bad experience, such as encountering a snake on a hike or a partner with bad breath in a dancing class, may believe that they will always have similar bad experiences. Instead of giving the activity another try or trying another activity, they write off any kind of exercise. To fight the tendency to globalize, try to figure out what caused the bad experience and how you can adapt either yourself or the activity for greater enjoyment.

- Perhaps the greatest barrier to change is lack of time, but did you know that the average American over age 2 watches 34 hours of live television per week and 3 to 6 hours of taped or recorded programming? And Americans over age 65 watch, on average, 48 hours of television per week. The fact is that we have time, but we choose to spend it on non-fitness activities.
  - If you really can't give up your TV watching, then put it to work for you. Put your treadmill or elliptical in front of your television. If you're not quite ready to put exercise equipment in your living room, do squats, sit-ups, and stretches during commercials. If you watch 2 hours of television every evening, you could get in 28 minutes of exercise!

  - You should also put fitness on your schedule and treat it as seriously as you would a meeting or an appointment. Consider it self-care and a valuable part of your day. If it helps you stay more committed, make a date with a friend or family member to walk or go to the gym after work.

  - Remember that small blocks of time add up. Instead of looking for 30-minute blocks of time during the day, try to find 5 or 10 minutes. If a meeting ends 10 minutes early, walk a loop around your office building. Stretch for 5 minutes while your coffee finishes brewing or do 1 minute of resistance exercises while you wait for your toast.

- A final barrier to change is the idea of risk complacency and the illusion of invincibility—the belief that disease happens to other people. Many younger people have this attitude, but the illusion becomes harder to maintain as we get older. We start to feel the effects of our own poor choices, and we watch as our parents pass away or our friends and peers deal with illness. Ultimately, we start to realize that disease can affect everyone.
  - Unfortunately, this shift in perspective can lead to another barrier to change: a sense of indifference and helplessness. If we're all going to die anyway, why should we bother to change?

  - Of course, we all are going to die, but the choices we make can have a great deal of impact on the quality of the years we have.

Never Too Old to Start
- Scientists used to believe that the brain had a window for plasticity—for change in response to the environment—and that after a certain age, we were less able to learn new things. This thinking led to the idea that only children can learn foreign languages to fluency or that to really learn a sport or a musical instrument, you have to start as a child.

- Recent neuroscience, however, has fundamentally changed our understanding of the human brain and its capacity for change and evolution. Neuroscience and its ability to map brains has helped us understand that our brains our constantly growing and reacting to the environment throughout the lifespan.
  - One interesting study compared London bus drivers, who drive fixed routes, with London taxi drivers, who might drive anywhere on London's 25,000 streets. The taxi drivers' brains actually showed growth in a part of the brain related to knowledge of maps.

○ Another study found that medical school students showed changes in the parts of the brain related to memory after studying for and completing their exams.

○ One study demonstrated that even older adults with cognitive impairment have brain plasticity. After 6 weeks of a deliberate memory-training program, they improved their performance on memory tasks by 33%, and magnetic resonance imaging (MRI) scans showed increased activity in their brains.

• These types of studies confirm that we can make changes later in life, and such changes can make a difference in quality of life for our remaining years.

• Motivations may be different for each of us; one person may see the need to fight a bad genetic history; another may want to play with a grandchild in the park or take an outdoor-oriented vacation. Identifying your motivation is an important first step to improving your fitness; take some time to find that spark that will get you up and moving.

Suggested Reading

Bandura, *Self-Efficacy*.

Prochaska, Norcross, and DiClemente, *Changing for Good*.

Activities and Assignments

In your journal, assess where you are in the stages of change: precontemplation, contemplation, preparation, action, or maintenance. What will help you move forward?

What are your personal motivators for fitness? Brainstorm as many motivations for fitness as you can.

Getting and Staying Motivated
Lecture 2—Transcript

We're smart people, but smart isn't enough. Knowing what we should do is not enough to make us do it. Though most of us know the benefits of physical activity, few of us are sufficiently active. Research shows that more than 80 percent of adults do not meet minimal guidelines for recommended physical activity, and as many as 34 percent of older adults are completely inactive.

So what is it that gets us moving? A fundamental component is motivation, which is the desire and will to do something. Motivation is affected by our locus of control, which is our sense of internal versus external control. We discussed locus of control in our first lecture, and how people with internal locus of control are healthier. This is because if you have an internal locus of control, you believe that you have the power to change things and to have an impact on outcomes. For your health, this is particularly important, because an internal locus of control means that you are more likely to engage in health-promoting behaviors, specifically because you believe that you have the power to change your health and impact your health outcomes.

Research also shows that our capacity for imagination can help us make better decisions. I'm not talking about our ability to imagine stories or create art, but rather our capacity to imagine ourselves in other situations and scenarios. For instance, if you can imagine yourself as an older adult and contemplate what that will mean, you are more likely to make good decisions to prepare yourself for that outcome. People who can imagine themselves as older adults make better decisions to support healthy aging, even save more money for retirement. There are even websites that will allow you to upload a photograph of yourself, and then electronically age yourself, so that you can see what you'll look when you are older. This helps you more concretely connect to your older imagined self, and then make the right decisions for your health and well-being in a few decades.

Let's talk more about motivation. One theory of motivation is the Transtheoretical Model of Behavior Change, also called the Stages of Change Theory. This theory holds that when faced with a potential change, our motivation falls in one of six stages: precontemplation, contemplation, preparation, action, maintenance, and termination. Let's walk through each of these stages, using a smoker as an example to illustrate what each stage looks like.

Precontemplation can be thought of as not ready for change. Someone who is in precontemplation does not intend to take action or make a change, and may not even be aware that their behavior is problematic. A smoker in precontemplation has no intention of quitting smoking. If his spouse doesn't like smoke and doesn't allow him to smoke in the house, he views that as his spouse's problem; he may cooperate and restrict smoking to the outside of the house to placate his wife, but he doesn't consider that a reason to stop smoking.

An individual in contemplation is getting ready for change; this is someone who is starting to recognize that they may have a problem. They are spending cognitive energy looking at the pros and cons of the behavior to determine whether they want to make a change. Perhaps the smoker has a new grandchild, and the grandchild's pediatrician has provided information about the dangers of third-hand smoke, and how the lingering smoke on his clothes and hands can put the new baby at a higher risk for asthma and allergies. So he's still smoking, but he is careful to wash his hands, to change his clothes before holding the baby, and he's starting to think that smoking has a downside. It might be more trouble than it's worth.

An individual who moves to preparation is actually intending to take action in the immediate future. This individual may even begin to make small steps toward the change. Our smoker has decided that he should quit smoking. He has made an appointment at a smoking cessation clinic. He has bought a few packs of nicotine gum and a box of patches. He is still smoking, but he is taking the preparatory steps toward making a change.

When the individual actually begins to make the change, through specific, overt behavior modifications towards a new healthy behavior, they have moved into the action phase. In action, our smoker has stopped smoking. He is wearing the patch, and chewing nicotine gum; he hasn't smoked a cigarette in several days. He is also assessing his life and figuring out how to better support the change. For instance, he has had his carpets and the upholstered furniture in his house professionally steam cleaned, and has also had the interior of his car steam cleaned. With help from the smoking cessation clinic, he is trying self-hypnosis and meditation to work through stress, instead of smoking.

Once he has been a nonsmoker for several months successfully, he will have moved to the maintenance phase. This is when an individual has successfully maintained the new, healthy behavior for a substantive period of time. They are still working actively to prevent a relapse. At some point, maintenance moves to termination; this is the stage in which the individual is no longer tempted to relapse. Some psychologists believe that termination occurs when you have successfully maintained the behavior for at least one year.

However, for some behaviors, such as addiction to drugs or alcohol or smoking, relapse can occur even after years of maintenance. Because of this, some psychologists believe that a changed individual is always in maintenance and will always have to actively work to maintain the healthy behavior. It may be that some individuals are more prone to relapse than others, so it's important to be aware of your own tendencies when making a behavior change, so that you can set yourself up for success.

So, think about your own fitness and wellness, and assess where you are. You're at least in contemplation – you're watching the course, so you're at least thinking about becoming more fit and more healthy. Even if you didn't buy the DVD yourself and you received it as a gift, you're contemplating the idea of change enough to actually put the DVD in and press play.

It's important for you to think about what phase you are in and assess your motivation, because motivation is personal. I can tell you my motivation, but my motivation won't get you active. Let me share a few examples.

I have a good friend Joe. He's a wonderful ballroom dancer. I met Joe when he was in his 80s, and a regular yoga student in one of my yoga classes. In his 80s, Joe was fit and strong and had great balance, and a motivator for him was how much he loves to dance. He continues to dance regularly, a decade later. It's great exercise, but that's not why he does it. To Joe, dancing is about the music, the connection with friends, getting out and interacting with other people. As he has gotten older, he has to rest more, so sometimes he has to sit out every other dance, but he's still dancing.

We have another dear family friend named Jerry, who is a master's swimmer. He is competitive at the national level. Whenever I see Jerry I ask how his swimming is, and he jokes with me that he is going to win first place one day at nationals, because he's going to outlive everybody else. For Jerry, that's a motivator, the idea that he's staying healthy and will endure.

Another aspect of motivation is the things that get in the way of us doing what we set out to do. These are called barriers to change. Let's talk through common barriers to change, and how we can overcome them.

Procrastination is a common barrier to change. This is: I'll do it later; I'll do it tomorrow, or next week, or next month, when I get new shoes, once I've lost a few pounds and I feel more comfortable going to the gym. But we keep putting things off to another time. In many cases, procrastination may be connected to our fear of perfection. We worry that we aren't good enough, we can't do it well enough, so we give up before we even try. But generally in life, and certainly when we are talking about our health, good enough really is good enough. It's better to accept the good enough than to keep waiting for perfect. Voltaire said it: "The best is the enemy of the good." Do what you can do today; do something, do anything, just get started.

Instant gratification is another barrier to change. You mean well; you want to make healthy choices, but it's been a long day, and you're tired, and it's more fun to watch TV, or have a snack, or read a book, or take a nap. So we choose the thing that seems like it will feel good now. The challenge, though, is we don't always know what really will make us feel good. Think about it, when you've let yourself lounge on the couch with too much junk TV and too much junk food. Do you even remember how the food tasted? Did you actually feel good doing that, or did you end up feeling more tired and kind of sick to your stomach by the end of it?

Remember that easy is not the same thing as gratifying. Yes, it may take a little push to get you out the door for a walk in the fresh air, but once you're walking, you will feel good from the fresh air, the activity, and the sunshine.

Another barrier to change are preconditioned beliefs. These can get in our way. Maybe you say to yourself, "I'm not an athlete." Says who? Just because you didn't play sports in high school or college? Your 18-year-old self does not define who you are today.

This is a barrier to change I've have often heard in my older adult fitness classes is. Sometimes I would hear from older women in class, "It's not ladylike. I don't want to sweat." I like to challenge that one because why not? You can be elegant and fit. For all of her activity, my grandmother never rode a bicycle. She didn't learn how when she was young, and when she was older she insisted that women couldn't ride bikes because it wasn't ladylike. We lived in Germany when I was a teenager, and all of my grandmother's German friends did ride bikes, even while wearing dresses and skirts. Somehow, in spite of that evidence to the contrary, she couldn't break through her preconditioned belief that riding a bicycle was not ladylike.

So ask yourself, what preconditioned beliefs are limiting me? What evidence can I find that I might be wrong, so that I can try something new? For instance, perhaps you are worried that you could hurt yourself and that it would be worse to be hurt than to be out of shape. You can challenge that. You can make fitness choices that are gentle, that have a low potential for risk. Skip the scary strenuous things like skydiving and contact sports. You're unlikely to get hurt going for a stroll on the sidewalk in your neighborhood, and if you're increasing the bone mass in your hips and lower spine with your walk, you're actually reducing your risk of injury.

Another common belief is that a little exercise won't make a difference anyway, so why bother? The truth is that a little bit of exercise actually will make a difference. A large study published in 2008 in the *British Journal of Sports Medicine* reported that just 20 minutes of physical exercise per week is sufficient to promote mental health. Going for a moderate walk for 30 minutes five times per week is enough exercise to significantly reduce your risk of dying prematurely. So a little exercise will actually make a big difference. Doing more brings additional benefits – but any additional fitness you do will improve your health and well-being.

Another common barrier to change is the fear of discomfort: Exercise hurts. Exercise makes me tired. I could injure myself. That can be true; it's true that exercise can be uncomfortable. It can make you tired. But if you choose an exercise program that is right for your body, your abilities, and your interests, uncomfortable isn't the same as pain. I don't want you to push so that you injure yourself, but I do want you to work through your sense of discomfort and set new expectations for yourself. You may be tired after a workout, but when you're tired from a workout, you'll discover that you sleep so much better and feel much more rested the next day. If you've ever suffer from insomnia and have a difficult time turning your mind off at night, the physical weariness that can come from a good workout will help you go to sleep instead of tossing and turning.

Let's develop new frameworks together. The reality for most of us is that the injuries and surgeries that we experience as we get older often lead to chronic pain. We have to adapt our expectations. We don't want pain; we don't want exercise that injures us, but some discomfort, some sense of muscle fatigue is normal and part of the process of becoming stronger and actually having less pain in the long run. You have to find that balance in yourself, and figure out where your perfect spot of challenge without pain is. We'll talk more about chronic pain and exercise in Lecture 10.

Another common barrier to change is globalizing. Maybe you had a bad experience last time, so you're worried that will always happen. Perhaps you have never tried a yoga class, and a friend pulls you into trying one, and the instructor has hairy armpits, and the mats are sweaty, and the incense makes you sneeze, so you decide "I'm never trying that yoga stuff again." Or you go to a ballroom dance class, and you get stuck dancing with that annoying partner with bad breath who keeps stepping on your toes and telling you that you're the one moving the wrong way. Or you finally lace up your shoes and you go for a hike on a trail near your neighborhood, and right away, you have to detour because of a massive anthill and there's a bull snake in your path and it's just overwhelming.

So you could just quit. You could write it off. Say yoga or dancing or hiking or whatever is not for you. Or you could give it another try. Or try another activity. Talk to other people who enjoy the activity to find out what they are doing differently. For instance, the yoga class—there are over 100 different styles of yoga taught in the U.S., ranging across the spectrum from new age to rehabilitative. A different style and a different teacher will be a drastically different experience. We'll talk more about yoga in Lecture 6, when we discuss mindful fitness.

The dance class: If you don't have your own partner and you're not willing to risk the roll of the dice, look for a partner-free type of dance like line dancing or tap dancing. Or, look for a studio that requires everyone to rotate around the room during a lesson; then you'll never be stuck with any one partner for more than a few minutes. Of course, the downside of the rotating is that if you do meet a great partner, you still only get to dance for a few minutes. For the hike, maybe try a different trail, or start with a walk in the park, or invest in a good pair of hiking shoes that will protect you from whatever random critters you encounter. The point is, give it another try.

It might also be that there is something truly wrong, and your discomfort and bad experience was indicative of something else. When my mother was a captain in the Army, she had chronic leg pain every time she ran. She had to run every day, and this was the era when you had to run in combat boots. She was convinced that there was something wrong with her, and that she just wasn't a runner because everyone else seemed to enjoy running. She had to run, the Army required it; she just decided that running was awful but she'd work through it. Finally, she was describing her constant chronic shin pain to one medical officer, who referred for some additional exams. They discovered she had tumors growing in the front bones of both of her shins. No wonder she had pain. In that case discomfort was an indicator of a health condition, not a reflection of the activity.

That's my point: Don't allow one bad experience to globalize your perception of physical activity. Try to figure out what's causing the bad experience, and how you can adapt either yourself or the experience into something you enjoy.

Another common barrier to changes is a lack of time. The idea that I'm too busy, work is more important, I don't have 30 minutes, I don't have 15 minutes. But ask yourself: Really? Do I really not have 15 minutes to go out for a walk after dinner or maybe do a few stretching exercises before bed? Did you know that the average America over age two watches 34 hours of live television per week, and an additional three to six hours of taped or recorded programming, plus spends another 5 hours a week just surfing the internet? Americans over the age of 65 watch, on average, 48 hours of television a week. That's seven hours a day!

I'm telling you this to make the point that we have time. We are just choosing to spend it in non-fitness activities.

Another place to shift your perspective: If you really can't give up your TV watching, put it to work for you. Try putting your treadmill or elliptical in front of your television. You can even buy energy-generating fitness equipment; you hook your TV up to your treadmill, and it only runs when you're creating energy with your movement! Yes, I know your living room will look unusual will a treadmill sitting in front of your television, but a pretty sofa is not going to help you live longer. Maybe you're not ready for exercise equipment in your living room; that's OK. You can still put your TV time to productive use. The average 30-minute television show is only 23 minutes of programming, with 7 minutes of advertising per half-hour. Put those commercial minutes to good use; do do some squats, do some sit-ups, do some stretches. Walk around your couch. With two hours of television watching in an evening, the commercial breaks would add up to 28 minutes of exercise!

You should also put fitness on your schedule and treat it as seriously as you would a meeting or an appointment. Consider it self-care, a valuable part of your day. If it helps you stay more committed, make it a commitment to a friend or family member. Make a date to walk or go to the gym with a friend after work, put it on your calendar, and then show up so that you don't let your friend down.

Remember that small blocks of time add up. So don't start out trying to find 30 minutes. Look for 5 minutes or and 10 minutes; if a meeting ends 10 minutes early, can you walk a loop around your building? Can you stretch for 5 minutes while your coffee finishes brewing? Can you do 1 minute of resistance exercises while you wait for your toast? We'll talk more in Lecture 5 about how to build physical activity into your life through activities of daily living, but the main point is to remember to look for the pockets of time that you already have.

Another common barrier to changes is the idea of risk complacency and an illusion of invincibility. This is the idea that disease happens to other people, I have good genes, I don't need to worry. So I can eat whatever I want, stay up as late as I want, drink as much as I want. This is common when we're younger. It becomes a harder illusion to maintain, as we get older. First, we start to feel the effects of our poor choices more and more. The day after we eat too much or drink too much we feel sick. We stay up late one night, and instead of being able to sleep until noon the next day to recover, we still wake up early with aching backs or hips or shoulders.

Then, we start to see our parents pass away; friends and peers get cancer, deal with high blood pressure, and have strokes. We have our own health scares, and hold our spouses' hands as they go in for surgeries. We start to realize that disease doesn't just happen to other people. Unfortunately, this shift in perspective can lead to another barrier to change: a sense of Indifference and helplessness.

This can happen if you start to feel like aging just happens, there is nothing I can do, so why bother, we're all going to die. And it's true. We are all getting older. We are all going to die someday. But the choices you make have an impact on a lot of years in the middle. True, there is always risk; even healthy people who make good decisions can end up in car accidents or have other tragedies occur. But the odds for a healthy life for as long as possible fall more on your side if you are making good, healthy decisions. It may be that you want to make good healthy decisions, but you think you're too old to start. Let's take a look at a couple of examples that disprove that notion.

Scientists used to believe that the brain had a window for plasticity, for change in response to our environment, and that after a certain age we were less able to learn new things. This led to the idea that only children can learn foreign languages to fluency, or that you have to start a sport or a musical instrument as a child to ever really learn them. When I was an undergraduate psychology major, I was taught that as we got older, the synaptic connections in our brain died, and this led to inevitable declines in performance. But neuroscience research has fundamentally changed our understanding of the human brain and its capacity for change and evolution. Neuroscience and its ability to map brains has helped us to understand that our brains are constantly growing and reacting to our environment throughout the lifespan.

For instance, one interesting study compared London bus drivers, who drive fixed routes, with London taxi drivers, who might drive anywhere on London's 25,000 streets. The taxi-driver brains actually showed growth in a part of the brain related to the knowledge of maps. Another study found that medical school students showed changes in the parts of the brain related to memory after studying for and completing their exams. Another study demonstrated that even older adults with cognitive impairment have brain plasticity. After six weeks of a deliberate memory-training program, they had improved their performance on memory tasks by 33 percent and showed increased activity in the brain, according to MRI scans.

My grandmother was a type-2 insulin-dependent diabetic. I grew up with her giving herself insulin shots. When she was in her late 70s, with some good nutritional guidance, she was actually able to lose some weight and get off of insulin; she still had to take diabetic medication, but her blood sugar was much more stable through weight loss and appropriate food choices. Dr. Dean Ornish is a cardiologist famous for using whole-food-based diets based on fruits, vegetables, and whole grains to actually reverse heart disease. His lifestyle program over a five-year period has been shown to reduce the clogging of the arteries and reduce the risk of a cardiac event. My point is you can make a difference in your health. In fact, research shows that as much as 80 percent of our health outcomes are determined by our decisions and not by our genes. We can make choices later in life that make a difference in our quality of life for the rest of our years.

My motivation stems from my grandparents. They lived with my family throughout my childhood, and helped raise me. They were Midwestern farmers, cattle-ranchers, who ate steak and eggs for breakfast every day. My family genetic history is not so good. At 19, even though though I was a fit and active and a vegetarian, my cholesterol was 220. A few years later, my grandfather had a series of massive strokes that destroyed the frontal lobe of his brain. I spent a year in my early 20s helping my mother and grandmother take care of my grandfather; he couldn't remember our names. He needed help with basic tasks like eating and going to the bathroom. For me, changing an adult diaper on the grandfather I loved and who had helped raise me was a life-changing experience, and it brought home for me that the genetic deck id stacked against me. So for me, a primary motivator is to do my best to fight the genetics that I have.

I am intent on putting as many good decisions up against my genes as possible. But my motivation won't get you active. You need to identify your motivation, and your driving force. I'd like you to pull your journal out. First, write down the five stages of change: precontemplation, contemplation, preparation, action, and maintenance. I'd like you to spend some time thinking about what stage you are currently in. If you're still in contemplation, what will help you move forward to preparation and action? If you're in preparation, what else do you need to do to move into action? If you're already in action, what steps do you need to take to make this maintenance?

Then, think about your personal motivators. Brainstorm as many as you can. Why are you watching this course? Why do you want to get fit? Why do you want to be healthy? Are you about to have your first grandchild and you want to be able to play in the park? Climb up the stairs and slide down slides? Maybe your spouse has asked you to take dance lessons for years, and you want to be able to keep up? Maybe you're planning a vacation with family and friends, and you want to hike and kayak and be active with them.

In the next lecture, we'll talk about the fundamentals of self-care, and how you can make good supportive decisions about your sleep, stress management, and other aspects of your life, to promote your overall health and fitness. These activities also require you to be motivated to care of yourself. So think deeply about your motivations. Take some time and really reflect so that you can find that spark that is going to get you up and keep you moving.

Self-Care Fundamentals
Lecture 3

S elf-care has become a trendy term, and it may often be confused with the idea of indulgence or pampering. But self-care is not about getting a manicure or allowing yourself a glass of wine each night. Instead, it means choosing behaviors that help you balance the effects of the stressors of modern life. Self-care may include some indulgence and pampering if little luxuries help you feel more balanced, but even more vital for self-care are the core behaviors that really matter for our health. In this lecture, we'll focus on sleep, nutrition, mental exercise, and stress management.

The Importance of Sleep
- In modern American society, we tend to view sleep as a burden, an inconvenience that gets in the way of the activities we want to perform. Often, successful professionals brag about how little sleep they get; they are so competent that they don't need as much sleep as the rest of us. But that idea is a fiction. No one functions well on minimal sleep.

- If you think 5 or 6 hours of sleep a night is enough for you, science proves otherwise. After sleep deprivation, people experience noticeable changes in brain activity as measured by an electroencephalogram (EEG). Such changes affect you across the board, reducing your concentration, working memory, mathematical capacity, even logical reasoning.

- Among the first deficits that occur during sleep deprivation are those in logical reasoning and complex thought. One 2004 study from Harvard Medical School found that hospitals could reduce medical errors by as much as 36% by cutting doctors' work shifts to no more than 16 hours and their total work schedules to no more than 80 hours per week. Other research has found that the rate of errors in surgery goes up each hour over the course of a surgeon's day.

- Ongoing lack of sleep also has long-term effects. One interesting example is weight gain. One study found that people who sleep 4 hours or less per night are 73% more likely to be obese than normal sleepers. A longitudinal study conducted by researchers at Stanford University tracked the sleep habits and hormone levels of more than 1,000 people for 15 years. Hormones that are vital in managing appetite were directly related to how much sleep the participants got.
  - There was also a demonstrated relationship between sleep amounts and body mass index (BMI). Almost 75% of the study participants reported that they slept less than 8 hours per night, and the increases in body mass were proportional to the reduced sleep.

  - The biggest risk seems to occur for people who sleep less than 6 hours per night, while the ideal BMI seems to occur for people who sleep 8 hours per night.

- Sleeping less than 5 or 6 hours per night also increases risks for developing diabetes and coronary heart disease and affects mental health. When we look at the overall picture of healthy aging, sleep may determine just how many years of healthy aging we have. Large cross-sectional studies indicate that sleeping 5 hours or less per night increases mortality risk by about 15%.

Changing Your Sleep Habits
- The quality and quantity of sleep matter so much that even if you make no other change, if you start getting 8 hours of sleep per night, you will have better health, feel better mentally, and probably lose weight.

- To promote both more and better sleep in your life, fix a bedtime and a wake-up time and stick to them. Your body will get used to falling asleep and waking up at the same time each day. If possible, match your bedtime and wake-up time to natural daylight hours. You are better off sleeping 8 hours from 10 p.m. to 6 a.m. than from 2 a.m. to 10 a.m.

- Don't consume caffeine or alcohol 4 to 6 hours before your bedtime. Alcohol has the immediate effect of making you sleepy, but a few hours later, when your blood-alcohol levels decrease, a stimulant effect kicks in that will interfere with your sleep. You're better off having a glass of wine in the afternoon—as long as you're not driving—than drinking wine with dinner.

- Exercise regularly, but avoid exercise 2 hours before bedtime. The changes in body temperature that occur as a result of exercise can affect your sleep cycle. The exception to this rule is a gentle, relaxing exercise routine, such as a gentle yoga program, that may help you calm down and go to sleep. You can also try other relaxation strategies, such as deep breathing, meditation, or progressive relaxation (systematically tightening and relaxing the muscle groups in the body).

- Dedicate your bedroom to only two activities: sex and sleep. Keep your TV, laptop, and working papers elsewhere. You want your unconscious mind to associate your bed and bedroom with sleep. The bedroom should be comfortable, quiet, and cool—between 60° and 68°.

- Finally, establish a pre-sleep ritual to help you transition from day into sleep. Turn off your electronics—your phone, tablet reader, computer, and TV—an hour before bedtime. Take a warm bath or shower and then read a book in a different room before heading into your bedroom. Follow the same routine every night.

The Importance of Diet
- A fitness program should be accompanied by a well-balanced diet to support overall health and wellness. If you're getting enough sleep, managing your stress, and exercising regularly, but you live on fast food, you will not experience optimum fitness and health.

- A healthy, well-balanced diet built around whole natural foods, particularly fresh fruits and vegetables, is essential. Research continues to demonstrate that it's better to get your vitamins, minerals, and other nutrients from fresh foods than supplements.

- It's also important to drink plenty of fresh water to stay hydrated. Even when you're working out, unless you're sweating excessively or training for a marathon, water, not an expensive sport drink—is your best source of hydration.

Mental Exercise
- Research has demonstrated that there are changes, even declines, in certain components of cognitive function with normal aging. For instance, reaction time and working memory are both affected as part of the normal aging process. However, cognitive function during normal aging should be viewed as a zone of possible functioning, with the individual's personal decisions and health constraints influencing where he or she is within that zone.

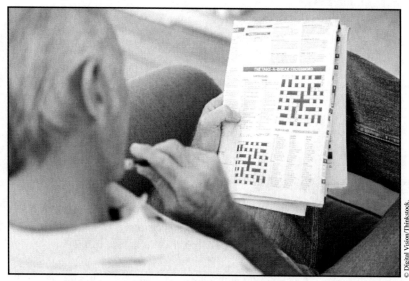

Just as you can make a difference in the way you age through physical exercise, so, too, can you make a difference in the way your brain ages through mental exercise.

- Neuroscience studies demonstrate that the older adult brain is still plastic; that is, it still has the potential for positive change. It's also true that older adults can leverage cognitive strategies to adapt to and even benefit from the changes that take place with aging. Older adults may approach learning and processing with new, different strategies, allowing them to continue to function effectively and efficiently.

- Mental exercise should be a part of your overall exercise program. Learning new things and challenging yourself with new adventures can actually stimulate the development of new neural connections to support brain functioning. Doing puzzles can engage both working and long-term memory and challenge your problem-solving skills. You can learn new patterns and new abilities by trying a new skill, such as taking up a musical instrument or learning a foreign language.

Stress Management
- The hormones related to chronic stress make you more prone to both short-term and long-term illness. Stress hormones also negatively affect your weight and your decision-making ability.

- Stress is defined as an automatic biological response to physiological, psychological, and sociological demands. The basics of stress boil down to a simple process:
  o A stressor occurs in the environment.

  o You perceive the stressor in a particular way (based on both other factors in the environment and your own personality, history, and knowledge).

  o If your perception is positive, the outcome is eustress, and you perceive the experience as positive.

  o If your perception is negative, the outcome is distress, and you perceive the experience as painful or uncomfortable.

Stress Reliever

Stand up and think back over all the stress and frustration you experienced during the day—all the times when you didn't get to do what you wanted to do, had to deal with someone who was being unpleasant, or got stuck in traffic or even mentally stuck.

Next, put your arms up over your head and shake them. Move as if you were a giant bowl of Jell-O. Shake your arms, your legs, and your head. Be silly, but move with every ounce of energy you have. Feel yourself pouring all your frustration and stress—all of your fight-or-flight responses—into your movement.

Now, stop and take a deep breath. How do you feel? Probably a little silly, but laughter is another great stress management technique. You should also feel more relaxed because you've gotten rid of the excess energy you accumulated by feeling stressed. Try this exercise at the end of any stressful day.

- Two people may experience the same environmental stressor very differently based on their perceptions. Some people perceive such events as riding a roller coaster or exploring a new city positively and feel eustress; others may perceive the same experiences negatively and feel distress.

The Impact of Stress

- When we talk about how stress affects us, it's helpful to look at three points in time: the immediate reaction, the acute reaction, and the chronic reaction.

- The immediate reaction to stress is commonly known as the "fight-or-flight" syndrome. When you perceive a stressor, you experience increased heart rate, blood pressure, respiration, and so on. These changes represent a primal response intended to help you either physically confront a danger or run away from it. If the stressor is physical and immediate, it is usually quickly resolved by the fight-or-flight reaction.

- In contrast, if the stressor is ongoing or can't be immediately resolved, then you begin to experience acute manifestations of stress, such as insomnia, digestive upset, emotional irritability, and so on.

- Both the immediate and acute reactions to stress can be uncomfortable, but stress levels only become problematic when they are chronic. When you experience ongoing stress over long periods of time, the constant roller coaster of the immediate stress responses combined with the slow wearing down of systems from acute reactions to stress lead to chronic health issues, such as hypertension, cardiac irritability, panic attacks, and more.

Optimal Stress Levels
- The optimal amount of stress is enough to provide motivation and energy but not so much that you burn out and wear down. How much stress is ideal is different for each of us, and having a sense of self-awareness to identify your ideal level of stress is one key aspect of managing stress.

- The psychological theory of the individual zone of optimal functioning (IZOF) states that we each have our own unique levels of ideal stress. The IZOF is often pictured as a bell-shaped curve. With a stress level that's too low, you experience low performance. As stress increases up to the IZOF, your performance increases. Once you reach the IZOF, additional stress decreases your performance.

- Once you know your preferred level of stress, you can use stress management techniques to support that level. Effective stress management requires becoming aware of events that commonly cause you stress; taking care of your health through a nutritious diet, sufficient sleep, and moderate exercise; using appropriate strategies, such as time management techniques, to prevent common stress-inducing situations; having a social support system; and preparing yourself to deal with stress through mental exercise and relaxation techniques.

- Healthy coping techniques for stress management include exercise; goal setting; time management and organization; reframing (viewing a situation from a different perspective); and breathing exercises, meditation, and progressive relaxation.

Suggested Reading

Anding, *Nutrition Made Clear*.

Epstein and Mardon, *The Harvard Medical School Guide to a Good Night's Sleep*.

Heller, *Secrets of Sleep Science*.

Sapolsky, *Stress and Your Body*.

———, *Why Zebras Don't Get Ulcers*.

Activities and Assignments

Assess your sleep quality and quantity. How much sleep are you getting per night? How do you feel with the current amount of sleep you get? Do you wake up rested? Do you feel groggy in the mornings, at midday, or at bedtime? What can you do to improve your sleep hygiene? Assess changes in your bedroom and your bedtime routine. What can you do to adjust your schedule to support the goal of getting 8 hours of sleep per night? What additional support or resources do you need to embrace the value of sleep in supporting your health?

What is your IZOF (individual zone of optimal functioning)? Over the next week, reflect at the end of each day on the stressors you experienced and how they affected the way you feel. Think about such stressors as lost items (your keys, cell phone, wallet), deadlines (at work or at home, such as paying bills on time), your own tardiness or the other tardiness of others, social interactions (parties, situations in which you meet new people, arguments or debates with friends or colleagues), and external factors (traffic, the line in the grocery store). How does each experience make you feel physically—tired or energized? Do you feel a knot in your stomach or a rush of excitement, a headache or a sense of clarity and purpose? What stressors support your performance and what stressors reduce your performance? Under what amount of stress do you perform at your best?

Think about opportunities you can find to experience eustress. What fun, new challenges could you try to have a eustress experience? You can start small, with something that is a little bit stressful but could be fun, such as a trip to a place you'd like to visit or the opportunity to learn a new language or musical instrument.

Self-Care Fundamentals
Lecture 3—Transcript

To be truly well, you have to take care of yourself. Self-care has become a trendy word, and you may have it jumbled together with ideas of indulgence and pampering. So let's start by talking about what self-care is, and how self-care is a foundational component of a healthy lifestyle. Self-care means choosing behaviors that help you balance the effects of the stressors of modern life. Pampering yourself may mean that you get manicures or pedicures or take regular vacations. Indulgence may mean that you let yourself have the chocolate or the wine because you deserve a break. Self-care means that you take care of your body, your mind, and your emotions. It means that you choose things that promote your wellness and that help you work through distress. That may well include some indulgence and pampering, if a massage every other week and a glass of wine with dinner help you to feel more balanced. Even more vital for self-care are the core behaviors that really matter for our health. In our discussion on self-care, we're going to focus on sleep, nutrition, mental exercise, and stress management.

Sleep is an interesting topic to discuss in our society, because we look at sleep, as a culture, as a burden, an unnecessary task we should do as little as possible, something that just gets in the way. Think about the number of people you know, successful professionals, who brag about how little sleep they get, as if it makes them stronger, braver, better people than the rest of us. They are so competent that they don't need sleep like the rest of us.

But that's a fiction. No one functions on minimal sleep. Minimal sleep compromises everyone's performance, health, and life. Even if you think you're functioning just fine on five or six hours of sleep a night, science proves otherwise. After sleep deprivation, there are noticeable changes in brain activity, as measured by electroencephalogram, or EEG. The changes are related to lower levels of alertness. Any time you have been awake beyond about 16 hours, an EEG will start to show changes in brain activity. And these changes impact you immediately, across the board, reducing your concentration, your working memory, your mathematical capacity, even your logical reasoning.

One of the first deficits that occur during sleep deprivation is in logical reasoning and complex thought. One 2004 study from Harvard Medical School found that hospitals could actually reduce medical errors by as much as 36 percent if doctor's work shifts were no more than 16 hours, and their total work schedule was no more than 80 hours per week. Other research has found that the rate of errors in surgery go up each hour over the course of a surgeon's day. So the next time you have surgery, you may want to ask your surgeon to schedule you at the start of her shift, and avoid a day where she was on call the night before.

An ongoing lack of sleep has a long-term impact. One interesting example is weight gain. One research study found that people who sleep four hours or less per night are 73 percent more likely to be obese than normal sleepers. A longitudinal study conducted by researchers at Stanford University tracked the sleep habits and hormone levels of over 1,000 people for 15 years. Hormones that are key in managing appetite were directly related to how much sleep the participants got.

So it's not surprising that there was also a demonstrated relationship between sleep amounts and body mass index. Almost 75 percent of the study sample reported that they slept less than eight hours per night, and the increases in body mass were proportional to the reduced sleep. The biggest risk seems to occur for people who sleep less than 6 hours per night. The ideal body mass seems to occur for people who sleep eight hours per night. In fact, sleep is so important for healthy weight management that some weight-loss programs have you focus on getting sufficient sleep before they address your diet and your exercise.

It's not just weight, though. Sleeping less than five hours per night increases your risk for developing diabetes. In one research study, when participants had their sleep reduced from eight to four hours, their bodies actually processed glucose more slowly. And the quality of sleep matters. Individuals with sleep apnea, a disorder that leads to problems breathing when sleeping, are at a higher risk for developing diabetes.

Sleep also affects your heart. One study with women found that women who slept less than six hours or more than nine hours a night had a greater risk for developing coronary heart disease. And in individuals who already have hypertension, just one night of sleep deprivation raises high blood pressure throughout the following day. Again, here as well, quality matters as much as quantity. People with untreated sleep apnea are more likely to develop hypertension and heart disease.

It probably comes as no surprise that sleep also matters for your mental health. In research studies, when healthy individuals were deprived of sleep or put on reduced sleep schedules, they reported feeling more sad, more stressed, more angry; they experienced lower levels of optimism and sociability. Is it any wonder that new parents often report that their marriages have declined in quality and that they're frustrated all the time, since nothing so dramatically reduces your sleep as the early years of parenthood? In those studies, once the participants went back to normal sleep schedules, their moods returned to normal.

When you look at the overall picture of healthy aging, sleep may determine just how many years of healthy aging you have. Large cross-sectional studies indicate that sleeping five hours or less per night increases your mortality risk by about 15 percent. Lack of sleep also puts your life at risk via accident. The Institute of Medicine estimates that drowsy driving is the primary cause of 20 percent of car crashes.

The quality and the quantity of your sleep matters so much, that even if you make no other change, if you start getting eight hours of sleep per night, you will have better health, feel better mentally, and probably even lose weight. So let's talk a little about strategies that promote both more and better sleep. Good sleep hygiene is key to supporting your health and fitness through sleep.

The first thing you should do: Fix a bedtime and a wake-up time and stick to it. Your body will get used to falling asleep and waking up at the same time each day. If you vary your wake-up time to sleep in on the weekends, sleep in no more than one hour so that you keep your body on schedule. If possible, match your bedtime and wake-up time to natural daylight hours. You are better off to sleep eight hours from 10 pm to 6 am than from 2 am to 10 am, or 10 am to 6 pm. Longitudinal studies of night-shift workers show that even those who manage to get sufficient sleep suffer additional chronic health impacts. Our bodies function better when we get sufficient sleep that is on schedule with the body's normal circadian rhythms.

To improve your sleep, also think about limiting caffeine. Your coffee in the morning is fine—in fact, some research shows that coffee has benefits for our health, mental health, and cognitive function—but espresso after dinner is a bad idea. Limit caffeine 4 to 6 hours before bedtime. You should also limit alcohol in the 4 to 6 hours before bedtime. It has an immediate effect of making you sleepy, but a few hours later as the blood alcohol levels reduce, there is a stimulant effect that wakes you up and interferes with your sleep. So, you're better off to have that glass of wine as an afternoon siesta, as long as you're not driving, than to drink wine with dinner.

To improve sleep, exercise regularly, but avoid exercise two hours before bedtime. The changes in body temperature that occur due to exercise can affect your sleep cycle. Your body gets warmer when you exercise; your body needs to be cooler to sleep. The one exception is gentle, relaxing exercises, since as a gentle yoga program, that might actually help you calm down, unwind, and go to sleep.

You can try other relaxation strategies; deep breathing, meditation, physical strategies like progressive relaxation. Progressive relaxation is a relaxation technique in which you systematically tighten and relax your muscle groups. This helps you to become aware of residual tension you may be holding without even realizing your stress. Try the progressive relaxation session in our active lectures right before bedtime, to help you relax and go to sleep.

You also need to set up your sleeping environment to support sleep. Dedicate your bedroom to only two things: sex and sleep. Keep your TV, your laptop, and your work, out of your bedroom. You want your unconscious mind to associate your bed and your bedroom with sleep. You also want to think about the environment of your bedroom. Your bed should be comfortable, quiet, and cool. Research indicates that if you are wearing light pajamas and using a light blanket, the ideal sleeping temperature is between 60 and 68 degrees.

You should also use a pre-sleep ritual, to help you transition from day into sleep. Turn off your electronics an hour before bedtime. That means all electronics: your phones, your tablet reader, your computer, your television—off and out of your bedroom. The glow from electronic devices can actually stimulate your brain to keep you awake. Take a warm bath or shower, use a favorite lotion. Try a scent like lavender, which promotes relaxation). Maybe read a book, an actual paper book, in a dim room, and then head to your cool, quiet bed. Do the same thing every night. The thing is that when it comes to bedtime, in our hearts, we are still little ones, and we crave consistent, comforting routines to allow us to settle peacefully off to sleep. So put yourself to sleep gently, so that you can truly sleep well.

A fitness program should be supported by a well-balanced diet, to support overall health and wellness. If you're getting sleep, managing your stress and exercising regularly, but you live on fast food, you are not going to experience optimum fitness and health. A healthy, well-balanced diet, built around whole natural foods, fresh fruits and vegetables, providing a balanced profile of vitamins, minerals, and other nutrients is key. Research continues to demonstrate that it's better to get those vitamin, minerals, and nutrients from fresh foods instead of supplements.

It's also important to drink plenty of fresh water so that you stay hydrated. Even when you're working out, unless you're sweating excessively or training for a marathon, water is your best source of hydration. You can actually skip those expensive sport drinks. In fact, if you do work out heavily, skim chocolate milk is a great post-workout drink, because it provides a nice balance of carbohydrates and protein to replenish your muscles. If you'd like additional supportive guidance about how to build your diet, The Great Courses offers a wonderful lecture series on nutrition that you can check out.

As we discussed in our first lecture, research has demonstrated that there are changes, even declines, in certain components of cognitive functioning with normal aging. For instance, reaction time and working memory are both impacted as part of the normal aging process. As you get older, you need to put more space between you and the car driving in front of you, so that you've got sufficient time to react. However, cognitive function during normal aging should be viewed as a zone of possible functioning, with the individual's personal decisions and health constraints influencing where he or she is within that zone. As we discussed in our last lecture, neuroscience studies demonstrate that the older adult brain is still plastic; that is, it still has the potential for positive change. We also know from psychological science that even if basic cognitive skills such as working memory capacity show inevitable decline with age, functional use of cognitive skills to achieve specific goals in specific situations does not have to decline. What that means is that though there are demonstrated changes in cognitive functioning with age, you can leverage cognitive strategies to adapt to and even benefit from these changes. Older adults may learn to approach learning and processing with new, different strategies, which allow older adults to continue to function effectively and efficiently.

So, just as you can make a difference in the way you age through physical exercise, you can make a difference in the way your brain ages through mental exercise. Mental exercise should be a part of your overall exercise program. Learning new things and challenging yourself with new adventures can actually stimulate the development of new neural connections to support brain functioning. Doing puzzles like crosswords and Sudoku can engage both working and long-term memory and challenge your problem-solving skills.

You can force yourself to learn new patterns and new abilities by trying a new skill. Take up a musical instrument; try a new sport; learn a foreign language. Research from North Carolina State University indicates that older adults who play video games, even occasionally, actually experience better mental health, so ask your kids or grandkids to try out their new game with you. It can be a great bonding experience. I still have very fond memories of learning how to play bowling and circus on my old Atari console with my grandpa. It may even enhance your hand-eye coordination and your spatial attention skills. One Italian study found that surgeons who regularly played the Nintendo Wii actually had better surgical skills! The bottom line is that your brain, like the rest of you, needs exercise, and you should be deliberate about planning new learning opportunities into your life, so that your brain and your awareness remain as healthy as the rest of you.

To support your goal of aging healthfully, there is another key aspect of self-care: stress management. Stress wears on your body. The hormones related to chronic stress make you more prone to both short-term and long-term illness. Stress hormones also affect your weight, making it harder to maintain a healthy weight. Stress hormones can also affect your decision-making ability, making it challenging for you to make good choices.

Let's talk more about what stress is, so that we can talk about how you manage it more effectively. Imagine you get on the elevator on the 19th floor of a building. The elevator jars, you hear the sound of the cable snapping, and then you drop more than 190 feet straight down. Physiologically, this is a stressful event, and your body will respond accordingly: your muscles will tense, your heart rate will surge, your awareness and senses will heighten, and your breathing rate will accelerate.

But as they say, stress is all in your head, because whether or not you perceive this as distress—the kind of negative stress that leaves your body hurting, your mind reeling, and your health impacted—or eustress, the kind of positive stress that leads to euphoria and subsequent relaxation, depends on what you think of the experience.

If you got on the elevator at your office building after a long day of work and you end up in this situation, it will clearly be a distress-provoking catastrophe. But if you stepped on the elevator after waiting in a long line at an amusement park for a "death drop" ride, you'll likely get off at the bottom feeling excited from the rush. Either way, it's the same physiological experience of dropping 190 feet, but the psychological perception fundamentally changes how you feel about the experience, and thus how you react to it.

Stress is defined as an automatic biological response to physiological, psychological, and sociological demands. As we just illustrated, you can boil the basics of stress down to a simple process: First, a stressor occurs in your environment. You perceive the stressor in a particular way (and this is based on both the other factors in the environment and the psychological aspects you bring to your environment, such as your personality, your history, and your knowledge). If your perception is positive, the outcome is eustress, and you perceive the experience as positive and wonderful. If your perception is negative, the outcome is distress, and you perceive the experience as painful, hurtful, and uncomfortable.

Two people will experience the same environmental situation very differently, based on their perception. Someone who loves running will experience a five-mile run as a eustress experience and finish on a classic runner's high. Someone who is not in physical shape for running will end the five miles feeling exhausted, worn out, and convinced that the runner's high is just a myth. The same is true for any experience: riding a roller coaster, riding a motor cycle, exploring a new city, going on a job interview, giving a speech, attending a party or concert or other social event. Some people will perceive each of those events positively and feel eustress; others will perceive the experience negatively and feel distress. The key to stress is your perception.

When we talk about how stress affects us, it's helpful to look at three points in time: the immediate reaction, the acute reaction, and the chronic reaction. The immediate reaction to stress is commonly known as the fight-or-flight syndrome. When you perceive a stressor, you will experience an increased heart rate, increased blood pressure, increased respiration, increased blood sugar, thickened blood, sharpened senses, prioritizing—which means blood supply increases to your heart and your large muscles (like your arms and legs) and decreases for other body parts, for instance the digestive system. You'll also have a secretion of adrenaline, and a secretion of endorphins

The reason for all of this is pretty basic; it really is about fight or flight. It's a primal response intended to help you either physically confront your foe, or else run away really fast. This is helpful if the stress you are facing is physically dangerous; if there's a mugger or if a car is driving too fast toward the crosswalk, that fight or flight is really going to protect you.

If the stress is physical and immediate, you will use your fight or flight to quickly resolve it and the manifestations of the stressor will also resolve. If the stressor is either something that continues or something that you can't immediately shake off, then you will begin to experience acute manifestations of stress. For instance, suppose you've got a big deadline coming up at work; you're putting in a few extra hours for a few days, you might find yourself experiencing: insomnia; digestive upset; emotional irritability, where you're feeling moody, sensitive, angry; you might have some difficulty concentrating; you might be forgetful.

Both the immediate and acute reactions to stress can be uncomfortable, but our stress levels only become problematic when they become chronic. When we experience ongoing stress over long periods of time, then the constant up-and-down roller coaster of the immediate stress responses, combined with the slow wearing down of our system from the acute reactions to stress, leads to chronic health issues. Chronic stress leads to health conditions like hypertension, cardiac irritability (which means we have a higher risk of heart disease). It can make us prone to panic attacks and other psychological disorders. It can actually decrease immune cell function, which makes you have an increased susceptibility to germs and infection. It can also lead to an excessive level of cortisol, which also compromises the immune system and also potentially increases weight gain.

You want some stress, because stress includes the positive eustress experiences, and also provides some spark and motivation to work, to achieve, to challenge yourself. But with too much stress, your health and performance will suffer. So the million-dollar question is: How much stress do you need? The optimal amount of stress is enough stress to provide motivation and energy, but not so much stress that you burn out and wear down. How much stress is ideal is different for each of us, and having a sense of self-understanding and self-awareness to identify your ideal level of stress is one key aspect of managing your stress.

There's a psychological theory called the Individual Zone of Optimal Functioning, or the IZOF, and that states that we each have our own unique amount of ideal stress. The IZOF is often pictured as bell-shaped curve. You've got a low stress level, you also have low performance. As the stress increases up to the IZOF, your performance also increases. Once you've reached that Individual Zone of Optimal Functioning, any additional stress decreases your performance. So, my IZOF is different than yours.

As an assignment, for the next few weeks I'd like you to be really self-aware. Pay attention to how you feel in potentially stressful situations. If you're running up against a deadline at work, does it make it harder for you to work, or do you thrive on the energy and perform better? If you're late for an appointment, does it give you a knot of worry in your stomach, or do you get some energy and a bit of a hum in your blood? If you're in an argument with a colleague or a friend, does it give you a headache and make you want to go back to bed, or do you walk away feeling charged and ready to take on the world?

One IZOF isn't better than another; they're just different, and you won't function at your best until you have a sense of what your best level of stress is. It may also help for you to understand where your family and friends function best. If you realize that your spouse thrives on a higher stress level than you do, it may help you be more understanding as he is late for appointments, rushes around at the last minute on projects, and gets charged up with debates over the news.

In contrast, if you're the high-stress-loving spouse but your partner functions best at a lower level of stress, it may help you to be supportive of her need to leave early, plan ahead, and avoid heated arguments. Stress management requires that you understand your own ideal level of stress, and then how to use stress management techniques to support your body in appropriately adapting to stress. Once you know what your preferred amount of stress is, the trick is using stress management techniques to support that level. Effective stress management requires several things. First, becoming aware of events that are your most common stressors, so that you can appropriately prepare for the stressors that affect you. You need to take care of your health, through healthy diet, sufficient sleep, and moderate exercise, so that your body is physically more able to adapt to and recover from stress. You might think about organizational strategies, time management techniques, things that will help you to prevent common stress-inducing situations. You also want to have a social support system, including family and friends, and to prepare yourself through mental exercise and relaxation techniques to better deal with stress.

There are many strategies that people use for stress management. Some of these are unhealthy coping techniques, like drinking too much, using drugs, or avoidance, and in the long run they end up creating more stress than they resolve. But healthy coping techniques can go a long way towards supporting your health and wellness. Exercise in particular can be an effective stress management strategy, since it provides an appropriate release for all of the physiological energy that is created by the fight-or-flight response.

Let's try a fun, simple exercise for a minute. Stand up out of your chair. Take a minute and let yourself feel and be aware of all the stress and frustration from your day, all the places where you didn't get to do what you wanted, or had to deal with someone else being unpleasant, or you got stuck in traffic, or you got stuck in the elevator, or just plain felt stuck.

Put your arms up over your head, as if you were a giant bowl of jelly, just shake. Shake your arms and your legs and your head. Be silly and be funny but move move move move move with every ounce of energy you have. Keep moving; feel yourself pouring all of your frustration and stress, all of your fight or flight, into your movement. Imagine that you're using all the energy of your jelly pose to run away from a lion on the plains. Because that's why you get that pent-up energy with stress in the first place, let's put it to good physical use.

Now stop, pause, take a deep breath. How do you feel? Probably a little silly, but laughter is another great stress-management technique. Hopefully you also feel more relaxed, like you got the pent-up energy out. Try it in real time the next time you're feeling stressed and you really need to get that energy out of your body.

Other healthy stress management techniques include things like goal setting. Goal setting is another healthy stress-management technique. We'll talk more about it in Lecture 7, when we return to the topic of motivation. Time management and organizational strategies can also be helpful for managing stress, particularly if you find yourself dealing with stressors like being late or losing your keys, or your spouse or children are late or lose things. You can also try environmental adaptations, which allow you to better structure your environment in ways to support your stress management. For instance, if you find your commute stressful, are there ways to make it a better experience? Can you try a different route? Carpool with a friend so that it becomes social time to talk? Can you listen to a Great Course so that it feels like your personal time to learn new things? We will talk more about the environment, and in particular, how you can adapt your environment to support your fitness, in our next lecture on motivation.

Reframing is another cognitive strategy that is particularly helpful for working through stressful situations. Reframing means that you try to view a situation through a different perspective, a different "picture frame." It's about looking for creative ways to find new opportunities in difficult circumstances, and looking for ways to build a positive outcome. Other effective stress-management strategies include breathing exercises, meditation, and progressive relaxation. We offer practice sessions of each of these in the active lectures. The Great Courses also has a lecture series focused on stress for those who want to more deeply understand the impacts of stress.

For the takeaways for this lecture, I'd like you to do a couple of things. I'd like you to think about how much sleep you're getting, and the quality of your sleep, and assess how you can improve both quantity and quality of sleep. What can you do to improve your sleep hygiene? How can you make changes in your life and your schedule so that you really commit to getting eight hours of sleep per night? Next, I'd like you to think about your stress, and identify your Individual Zone of Optimal Functioning, or your IZOF. How can you better organize your life so that you can live within your IZOF?

Finally, I'd like you to think about opportunities you can find for eustress. It seems to me that when we're young, we seek out eustress opportunities. We don't worry about the risks, the potential of falling or getting hurt. So we ride roller coasters; we leap off high dives; we go on dates for the thrill of the first kiss; we climb tall trees; we brave new adventures. But as we get older, we get more settled, we have more to lose, we become more risk averse, more risk avoidant. So what are the fun, new challenges you could try to have a eustress experience? You can start small, with something that is a little bit stressful, but which could be fun, and which is low-enough risk for you to not create anxiety. Maybe a trip to a place you'd like to visit, or learning a new language or instrument?

One great example of a eustress experience that we can continue to enjoy as we get older is making love. Cary Grant used to say that making love is the best form of exercise. And exercise is another important component of self-care, so lovemaking can help with both exercise and stress management! We will discuss the fundamentals of an exercise program in our next lecture, so that you have multiple tools to begin taking better care of yourself.

Fitness Fundamentals—Choose Your Activity
Lecture 4

In our last lecture, we talked about the fundamentals of self-care, of which physical activity and exercise are key components. In this lecture, we'll focus on how you can use physical activity and exercise to take better care of yourself. We'll begin with some foundational definitions of physical activity, physical fitness, and the key components of physical fitness. We'll also talk about the various types of exercise you need to incorporate into your routine and the components you need to include in your personal fitness plan.

Foundational Definitions

- Physical activity is movement by your skeletal muscles, movement that requires energy and produces health benefits. Physical activity is in contrast to physical exercise, which is physical activity that is planned, structured, and deliberate, intended to improve or maintain physical fitness. Physical fitness is the ability to meet the ordinary and unusual demands of daily life safely and effectively.

- Traditionally, when we talk about physical fitness, we talk about five key components: muscular strength, muscular endurance, cardiorespiratory endurance, flexibility, and body composition. In talking about fitness to support healthy aging, we add three additional aspects of fitness: balance and pelvic floor strength and endurance.

- Muscular strength is the ability to exert maximum force against resistance, that is, the ability to lift or move a heavy weight one time. Muscular endurance is the ability of a muscle to exert submaximal force repeatedly over time, that is, the ability to move or lift a light or moderate amount of weight multiple times.
  - Muscular endurance requires muscular strength. If you don't have a base level of strength, you won't be able to continuously move lighter items.

- Muscular strength and endurance are both specific and targeted. However, you can use strength-training exercises that target multiple muscles or groups of muscles to build your strength as efficiently as possible.

- Cardiorespiratory endurance reflects how the pulmonary, cardiovascular, and muscular systems work together during aerobic activities. Thus, cardiorespiratory endurance is the way in which your lungs, heart, and blood vessels collaborate to support you during constant movement. Without cardiorespiratory endurance, an individual's ability to move and function is severely limited.

- Flexibility is the range of motion you have at a joint or a group of joints—how much you can move that joint without causing injury. A lack of flexibility can be related to injury and can cause poor posture and chronic pain. Some research indicates that 80% of chronic low back pain in the United States is related to improper alignment of the vertebral column and pelvic girdle as a result of inflexible and weak muscles.

- Body composition refers to the fat and non-fat components of the body. BMI is the most widely used assessment of body mass and can be a rough estimate of health risk and mortality rate. A BMI between 22 and 25 indicates the lowest risk of chronic disease for both men and women.
  - Because fat tissue in the abdomen may be associated with higher risk for heart disease and diabetes, another simple measure of health risk using body composition is waist circumference.

  - A waist circumference above 40 inches for men and above 35 inches for women indicates increased disease risk.

- Balance is the ability to stay upright and remain in control of your body movement. When you have good balance, you are in control of your gait and have a sense of being sure on your feet. When your balanced is compromised, you are more likely to trip, lose your footing, or experience serious falls.

o Balance can be further divided into two types: static balance, which is the ability to stay upright while still, and dynamic balance, which is the ability to stay upright and remain in control while moving.

o Both types of balance are important, and both require that you have a strong core body and a good sense of body awareness.

- Pelvic floor strength and endurance, supporting voluntary control of the bladder and bowels, are a critical part of physical fitness as we get older. Even if you maintain all the other aspects of physical fitness, if you are no longer continent, your quality of life will suffer.

  o Urinary incontinence affects at least 10% to 30% of the population, and that's probably an underestimate. One study found that only half of individuals who had experienced urinary incontinence reported it to their physicians. Many women may think that urinary incontinence is a normal result of having babies or going through menopause.

  o Incontinence is related to poor ratings of one's own health, feelings of social isolation, depression, and impaired quality of life. It's also expensive; the annual estimated cost of urinary incontinence in the United States is $32 billion, or about $3,500 per person with incontinence.

  o It's important to understand that continence requires deliberate exercise, just like every other aspect of fitness. Older adults can take control in this area and support their own independence through exercise.

Types of Exercise
- To support overall physical fitness, your exercise program should include cardiovascular exercise, strength and resistance training, flexibility training, balance training, and pelvic floor exercises.

- Cardiovascular exercise is also called endurance or aerobic exercise. In this type of exercise, the body's large muscles move in a rhythmic manner for sustained periods of time, as in walking, jogging, swimming, biking, or dancing. Cardiovascular exercise increases your breathing and heart rate to improve the health of your heart, lungs, and circulatory system.

o   According to the American College of Sports Medicine (ACSM), you should do at least 30 minutes of moderate-intensity exercise 5 days per week. This can be broken up into three 10-minute blocks throughout the day. In fact, some research suggests that for certain health conditions, such as high blood pressure, three 10-minute blocks during the day may produce greater health benefits than one longer block. For even greater benefit, the ACSM recommends up to 60 minutes of cardiovascular exercise 5 days a week.

o   It takes 3 or more months of aerobic activity to see improvements in cardiorespiratory endurance—and you have to keep doing it to sustain the benefits.

•   Strength or resistance training includes exercises that cause your muscles to work or hold against an applied force or weight. Strength training increases both muscular strength and muscular endurance. You can do strength training using hand weights, resistance bands, strength training machines, or your own body weight.

o   Strength training is also important for your bones. As we age, bone density decreases, putting us at greater risk for fractures. Weight-bearing exercise provides support in maintaining bone density.

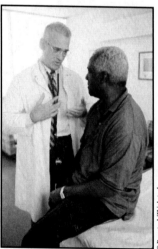

© Purestock/Thinkstock.

Older men, as well as older women, can also be at risk for osteoporosis; talk to your doctor if you have experienced a decrease in height.

o   The ACSM recommends that you do resistance training at least 2 days per week, with 8 to 10 exercises involving the major muscle groups. Aim for 8 to 12 repetitions of each exercise.

- Flexibility training refers to activities designed to preserve or extend range of motion around a joint. Flexibility training helps you stretch your muscles and stay limber so that you maintain independence in how you move. Deliberate stretching and such exercise programs as yoga and Tai Chi include flexibility training.
  o   The ACSM recommends that you do moderate-intensity stretching at least 2 days per week, using sustained, static stretches for each major muscle group.

  o   Static stretches are slow and controlled and make you less prone to injury. This is in contrast to the ballistic stretching (jumping and bouncing) you may have learned in high school gym class.

- Balance training refers to a combination of activities designed to increase lower-body and core-body strength and to reduce the likelihood of falling. Whole-body fitness programs, such as yoga, Tai Chi, and dance, include substantial balance work.

- Pelvic floor exercise is simple but critical to your overall fitness program.
  o   The first step is to identify your pelvic floor muscles. The next time you urinate, try to stop the flow of urine in midstream. The same contraction of muscles is used to do pelvic floor exercise.

  o   One simple pelvic floor exercise is to isolate the muscles of your pelvic floor, keeping your stomach, bottom, and thighs soft and relaxed. Then, lift up and contract your pelvic floor for a count of 5 and release.

Components of a Fitness Plan
- There are four key components of a fitness plan, and a simple acronym to remember them is FITT, meaning frequency (how

often), intensity (how hard), time (how long), type (what mode/type of exercise).

- Here's how the components translate: Let's say you commit to some simple cardiovascular exercise; you will walk (type) for 20 minutes (time) 3 times a week (frequency) at a gentle pace (intensity). After a month, you may decide to increase your walking to 5 times a week for 30 minutes at a faster pace. You may also add some strength and flexibility training; twice a week, you'll do chair yoga.

- As you work on your FITT plan, be realistic. Think about the types of activities you would enjoy, the activities your life will currently support, and how you can use the principles of FITT to start building physical fitness. What matters is that you craft a plan that works for you.

Suggested Reading

American College of Sports Medicine, ed., *ACSM's Complete Guide to Fitness and Health*.

———, http://www.acsm.org/.

Brill, *Functional Fitness for Older Adults*.

Activities and Assignments

Assess your health risk via body composition:
- Determine your BMI using the calculator available at: http://www. cdc.gov/healthyweight/assessing/bmi/adult_bmi/english_bmi_ calculator/bmi_calculator.html.

- Measure your waist.

- Establish an initial fitness plan, using the principle of FITT.

	Frequency	Intensity	Time	Type
Cardiovascular exercise				
Strength and resistance training				
Flexibility training				
Balance training				
Pelvic floor exercise				

Think creatively: What activity are you already doing that you could leverage into exercise through a more deliberate approach?

Fitness Fundamentals—Choose Your Activity
Lecture 4—Transcript

In our last lecture, we talked about the fundamentals of self-care. Physical activity and exercise are a key component of self-care. We will focus this lecture on how you can use physical activity and exercise to take better care of yourself. Let's start with a few foundational definitions.

Physical activity is movement by your skeletal muscles—movement that requires energy and produces health benefits. This is in contrast to physical exercise, which is physical activity that is planned, structured, and deliberate, intended to improve or maintain physical fitness. Physical fitness is the ability to meet the ordinary and unusual demands of daily life safely and effectively.

Let's think about what that means, the ordinary and unusual demands of daily life. Ordinary things like getting dressed in the morning, loading your groceries into the trunk of your car, and then carrying them into your kitchen, reaching a cereal box from a top shelf. Those are all ordinary things that require you to be able to lift and tote and move. Unusual demands are things like having to jump out of a crosswalk when a car comes a little too fast, or catch the arm of a friend if she starts to slip.

You can use physical activity to support physical fitness. You don't have to get into the gym—you can go for walks, lift your grandchildren, stretch in bed before you wake up. There are so many activities you can do as part of your daily life to support your physical fitness and your overall health.

Traditionally, when we talk about physical fitness, we talk about five key components: muscular strength, muscular endurance, cardiorespiratory endurance, flexibility, and body composition. Since we are talking about fitness to support healthy aging, we are going to add three additional key aspects of fitness: balance, pelvic floor strength, and pelvic floor endurance. Let's define each of the components of physical fitness.

We'll start with muscular strength and muscular endurance. Muscular strength is the ability to exert maximum force against resistance—your ability to lift or move a lot of weight one time. Muscular endurance is the ability of a muscle to exert submaximal force repeatedly over time—your ability to move or lift a light or moderate amount of weight multiple times. To use a simple example to contrast the difference, muscular strength is being able to move one heavy box, and muscular endurance is being able to carry several grocery bags back and forth from your garage to the kitchen. Muscular endurance requires muscular strength: If you don't have a base level of strength, you won't be able to continuously move lighter items.

Muscular strength and endurance are both specific and targeted. Strength in one muscle does not mean you will have strength in another muscle. However, you can use strength-training exercises that target multiple muscles or groups of muscles to build your strength as efficiently as possible. We'll focus on this kind of strength training in the Foundational Fitness workout.

Cardiorespiratory endurance reflects how the pulmonary, cardiovascular, and muscular systems work together during aerobic activities. So cardiorespiratory endurance is the way in which your lungs, your heart, and your blood vessels collaborate to support you during constant movement. *Aerobic* means "with oxygen," and aerobic exercise is the type of exercise that occurs when you maintain movement over time; for instance, walking, swimming, biking, and running. This is in contrast to anaerobic exercise, which is generally higher intensity in a very short time period. For instance, running a mile is aerobic exercise; it's repetitive over a longer period of time. But running a 100-meter dash in anaerobic—very high intensity, short period of time. Cardiorespiratory endurance may be one of the most fundamental components of fitness, because it allows us to do house and yard work, walk across a parking lot, or climb a flight of stairs. Without cardiorespiratory endurance, our ability to move and function is severely limited.

Flexibility is the range of motion that you have at a joint or a group of joints. It's how much you can move that joint without causing injury. Flexibility is important because a lack of flexibility can be related to injury. It can also cause poor posture and chronic pain. Some research indicates that as much as 80 percent of chronic low back pain in the US is related to improper alignment of the vertebral column and pelvic girdle, due to inflexible and weak muscles. Lack of flexibility in the chest and lack of strength in the back can cause a dowager's hump in older women. Chest stretches and back strengthening exercises are key for helping you maintain good posture and prevent back pain.

Let's review a few simple exercises that you can do at any time to open up your chest. These are great exercises to do throughout your day, particularly whenever you notice your posture caving in. One simple exercise is called the goal post. So, nice posture, either standing or sitting. Sit up nice and tall or stand up nice and tall. Arms are out wide, elbow to shoulder's a nice straight line. Fingers are spread wide and you're going to just pull back through the elbows, lifting and pulling so that you're opening up your chest, pulling the muscles of the back together, pulling the shoulder blades together. You're strengthening the muscles of the middle of the back; you're opening up the chest. This is a great stretch for the chest, a great strengthener for the middle of the back. It'll help you to feel nice and open. You can also do this lying down, either on the bed or on the floor. Just relax your arms out to the side in this posture. Relax that way for 10 or 15 minutes to really allow your body to relax into a chest opener, a really nice stretch.

Another simple thing to do: hands behind head. Interlace your fingers, bringing your hands behind your head. Pull out through the elbows. Lift up through the chin. You'll feel the strength in the muscles in your back pulling together at a higher point in your back than with goalpost. Pulling out, opening the chest, strengthening the back. Nice stretch here. Again, you can do this seated or standing. Then relax that.

Another one to try: fingers interlaced behind your back. You're lifting your chest, bringing your hands together, fingers interlaced. Lift your chest and chin, opening the front. If you're feeling comfortable here you can actually lift the arms up behind you to add some further stretch across the shoulders, really opening up the front of your body. Those are great stretches to do every day, proactively to stretch your chest, strengthen your back, but also great to do when you feel your posture starting to scrunch—if you're typing at your keyboard all day, or you're driving a long drive and your shoulders are starting to slump forward, great way to expand and open the chest.

Another component of fitness is body composition. Body composition means the fat and non-fat components of the body. A simple way to assess body composition is through Body Mass Index (or BMI). BMI is the most widely used assessment of body mass, and it can be a rough estimate of health risk and mortality rate.

A BMI between 22 and 25 indicates the lowest risk of chronic disease, for both men and women. All body-mass indicators have limitations, and one challenge with BMI is that it cannot distinguish between fat weight and muscle weight, so very muscular people may have high BMIs, which are therefore inaccurate in assessing their health risks.

Because fat tissue in the abdomen may be associated with higher risk for heart disease and diabetes, another simple measure of health risk using body composition is your waist circumference. A waist circumference above 40 inches for men, and above 35 inches for women, indicates increased disease risk because fat around the abdomen creates additional stress on the organs of the body. So get out your measuring tape and measure your waist and see where you are with that indicator as well.

Balance is your ability to stay upright and remain in control of your body movement. When you have good balance, you are in control of your gait, and have a sense of being sure on your feet. When your balanced is compromised, you are more likely to trip, to lose your footing, to experience serious falls. The health of your inner ear can affect your equilibrium and balance, as can your vision. If you wear bifocals or trifocals, that may actually affect how stable you feel on your feet. So balance is a multifaceted component of your health and fitness, and if you are experiencing challenges with your balance, it is a good idea to visit your doctor, and also to have your eyes and ears checked for health issues which are related to balance.

There are two types of balance: static balance, which is your ability to stay upright while still, and dynamic balance, which is your ability to stay upright and remain in control while moving. Both are important, and both require that you have a strong core body and a good sense of body awareness. Since falls are particularly dangerous as we get older, balance is a vital part of your physical fitness.

Let's talk about pelvic floor strength and pelvic floor endurance. These are a critical part of physical fitness as we get older. Because even if you have all the other aspects of physical fitness, if you are no longer continent, your quality of life will suffer. We are talking about the strength and endurance of your pelvic floor muscles to support voluntary control of your bladder and your bowels.

Urinary incontinence affects at least 10 to 30 percent of the population, but that's probably an underestimate. One study found that only half of those individuals who had experienced urinary incontinence reported it to their physician. Another study found that among women with urinary incontinence, as few as 14 to 38 percent talked to their doctor, and 46 percent of them waited until they had experienced incontinence for three years before talking to their doctor.

Women may think it's a normal part of what happens with aging because you've had babies; you've started to go through menopause perhaps. We write it off as a just being normal. And we don't talk about it, because we're embarrassed. But we should talk about it, because it matters. Incontinence is related to poor ratings of your own health, to feelings of social isolation, to depression, to impaired quality of life. It's also expensive: The annual estimated cost of urinary incontinences in the U.S. is $32 billion, about $3,500 per person with incontinence.

I have taught fitness classes to older adults in many different venues, and with many different areas of focus. But across the board, the best feedback and response I have gotten is from older adults to whom I have taught exercise programs that included pelvic floor exercise. I have heard from students who have been able to go back to church, an actually sit through an hour church service without having to run out to go to the bathroom. People who could go back to volunteering and not worry if a bathroom was going to be nearby. People who were able to spend time with friends and family, who could travel again because they were no longer worried about being away from the bathroom and no longer worried about having to carry along adult diapers and pads and wear them or use them.

If you've ever dribbled urine when you sneezed, or leaked a little when you laugh, jump, ran, or lift something heavy, then you've experienced a bout of incontinence, and pelvic floor exercise will help. If you go to the bathroom and you struggle to get started when you have to pee, or dribble a little bit when you're done, those are also symptoms of incontinence.

So, I'd like you to get over your embarrassment, because as part of this fitness program, we're going to talk about our pelvic floors. We're going to talk about how you can and should exercise your pelvic floor muscles to stay continent. The goal is for you to understand that continence requires deliberate exercise; you have to exercise the muscles of your pelvic floor, just like you exercise every other muscle of your body. It's another aspect of your fitness that you can take control of to support your independence and healthy aging through exercise. Since we're talking about incontinence I also want to make sure you are drinking enough water; sometimes, we consciously or unconsciously reduce our water intake because we think it will help with leaking, but the problem is it actually makes you prone to bladder infection, which makes incontinence more likely.

If you are experiencing ongoing issues, please do talk to your doctor; ask for a referral to an urologist or an uro-gynecologist. Incontinence can be related to other serious issues, and you'll want to make sure it's not a symptom of another health condition. However, if the first doctor you talk to writes it off as normal, talk to another doctor. Incontinence is not a normal part of aging, and you can regain control through deliberate exercise, and we're going to do those in this course.

To support overall physical fitness, your exercise program should include cardiovascular exercise, strength and resistance training, flexibility training, balance training, and pelvic floor exercises. Let's talk through each of those in a little more detail. Cardiovascular exercise is also called endurance exercise or aerobic activity. These are exercises in which the body's large muscles move in a rhythmic manner for sustained periods of time. Cardiovascular exercise increases your breathing and heart rate, to improve the health of your heart, lungs, and circulatory system. Cardiovascular exercise includes any activities that consistently keep your heart rate up, such as walking, jogging, swimming, biking, dancing, or sports where you stay in constant motion.

According to the American College of Sports Medicine, or the ACSM, you should do at least 30 minutes of moderate intensity cardiovascular exercise, five days per week. This can be broken up into three 10-minute blocks throughout the day. In fact, there is some research from Arizona State University that suggests that for certain health conditions, such as high blood pressure, three 10-minute walks throughout the day may actually produce greater health benefits than one longer block. In one study, blood pressure went down after each 10-minute walk, and even stayed down into the following day.

For even greater benefit, the ACSM recommends up to 60 minutes of cardiovascular exercise, five days per week. If you're doing vigorous activity, 20–30 minutes, three to five days per week may be sufficient. It takes three or more months of aerobic activity to see improvements in cardiorespiratory endurance, and then you have to keep doing it, to keep the benefits.

Strength training, also called resistance training, includes exercises that cause your muscles to work or hold against an applied force or weight. Strength training does exactly what it says: It helps you increase both your muscular strength and your muscular endurance. This maintains and improves your ability to stay independent, so that you can carry groceries, climb stairs, and safely complete other potentially strenuous activities of daily living. You can do strength training using hand weights, resistance bands, strength training machines, even your own body weight.

The type of strength training that we are talking about is not about looking like a movie star or someone in a bodybuilding competition. What we are talking about is about being able to open your own jars, put your own briefcase in the overhead bin, even stand up out of a chair without help. There are so many things we take for granted when we are young, but as we age, if we want to age healthfully and maintain our independence, we need to be deliberate about supporting and maintaining those aspects of physical fitness. Strength training becomes particularly important as we get older.

I'd like you to try an activity: The next time you are at a restaurant or café, take a look at how many people can sit down or stand up out of a chair without having to use their arms to support their weight. Then, keep an eye out for those magazine ads for chairs that physically lift you up out of the chair so that you don't have to use your own thighs. This is an area that most people start to demonstrate muscle loss, as they get older. But you can be deliberate about it. You can do squats and consciously focus on strengthening the muscles of your legs and your bottom.

Let's try it yourself. We're going to sit down in a chair without using hands for support for balance, and then stand up out of the chair without using your hands to push you up. Come to a chair, keep your hands out in front of you, and then try to sit down without falling into the chair. Then try again, to stand up without using your hands. As an experiment, contrast that. Put your hands down as you sit; push yourself up. Think about which way do you normally sit down and stand up—do you normally have to use your arms? Can you do it without your arms? Try building this into your day. It's a great simple exercise to strengthen your lower legs and low back. If every time you sit down you deliberately work to sit and stand just using the strength of your lower body, you'll be building that resistance training in throughout your day.

Strength training is also important for your bones. As we age, our bone density goes down, which puts us at a greater risk for fractures. Weight-bearing exercise helps support us in maintaining our bone density. Usually when we talk about osteoporosis, we think we're talking about women, but men are at risk as well. Do an honest self-assessment: measure your height. Don't just assume your height; actually measure it. How tall are you now? Have you lost any of the height you had in your late teens or early twenties? You probably still have your original height on your driver's license, but is it still accurate? Even a slight decrease in height can be an indicator of bone loss, and you should talk with your doctor about how do you better support the health of your bones.

The ACSM recommends that you do resistance training at least two days per week, with 8–10 exercises involving the major muscle groups, doing 8–12 repetitions of each exercise. The foundational fitness active session will walk you through some simple resistance exercises you can do at home using light hand weights and resistance bands.

Flexibility training refers to activities designed to preserve or extend range of motion around a joint. Flexibility training helps you to stretch your muscles and stay limber, so that you maintain independence in how you move. This is important as you age. Think about the things where you need flexibility—to fasten your own bra strap, zip your own dress, button your own shirt, reach down tie your own shoes, and reach packages in high cupboards. Deliberate stretching, and exercise programs such as yoga and tai chi all include flexibility training.

The ACSM recommends that at least two days per week you do moderate-intensity stretching, using sustained, static stretches for each major muscle group. Static stretches are slow and controlled; it's less prone for you to become injured. This is in contrast to ballistic stretching. That's the jumping/bouncing kind of stretching you might have learned in high school PE. In our course we have a chair yoga session, a Qigong session, and foundational fitness active sessions all designed to provide guidance on flexibility training.

Balance training is another component of fitness. Balance training refers to a combination of activities designed to increase lower-body and core-body strength and to reduce the likelihood of falling. Balance is so important as we get older because falls are a great risk for older adults. You have to be deliberate about your balance and doing balance exercise. You really can improve your balance through these exercises. Whole-body fitness programs like yoga, Tai Chi, and dance all focus on balance. They include substantial balance work. They strengthen the muscles of your core body, they strengthen your leg muscles, they improve your overall equilibrium. They also help you to feel steady on your feet, so that you are better able to recover from a slight trip, rather than falling. We will do balance exercises in several of our active sessions, again the yoga session, the Qigong session, and the core-body workouts.

Pelvic floor exercise is simple, but critical, to your overall fitness program. First, you'll need to learn how to actually recognize your pelvic floor muscles. So think about, have you ever tried to suppress gas in public? If so, you've deliberately contracted your pelvic floor. A simple way to learn how to isolate your pelvic floor muscles is with the what's called the stop test. The next time you're in the bathroom to urinate, try to stop the flow of urine midstream. That's the muscular movement you do when you're doing a pelvic floor exercise; it's that same contraction of your pelvic floor muscles. Only do this once or twice to identify that muscular movement. I don't want you to do it regularly—it can actually put you at risk for a bladder infection—but it's a great way to learn how to isolate the muscles of your pelvic floor.

Once you know how to isolate your pelvic floor, become deliberate about pelvic floor exercise. We're actually going to do an exercise right now. This is a simple exercise called the contract release. This is a basic pelvic floor lift. Focus your awareness on your pelvic muscle, your pelvic floor, isolating the muscles of your pelvic floor. Imagine that there's a hammock. You want to keep your stomach, your bottom, and your thighs soft and relaxed. If you're contracting your thighs or your bottom of your stomach, you're not isolating the pelvic floor. So keep those parts of your body soft and relaxed.

Focus on your pelvic floor and then lift up, as if you're pulling the muscle up inside your body and hold for 5, 4, 3, 2, 1 and then relax it. You want to relax for the same five-count that you contracted so that you allow the pelvic floor to really relax. Let's do one more. Lift it up and hold for 5, 4, 3, 2, 1 and relax. It should feel like a lifting.

We'll spend some more time doing pelvic floor exercises in the fitness fundamentals active lecture. You can do pelvic floor exercises as an integrated part of your fitness plan. You can also build them in throughout your day while you're standing in line, while you're driving in the car, while you're talking on the phone. Nobody can see you doing them, so it's a great exercise that you can do to strengthen your pelvic floor and improve your health throughout your whole day.

If you're ready, now, to be deliberate about your physical activity, let's discuss how we make a plan. There are four key components to any fitness plan, and a simple acronym to remember them is FITT: Frequency (or how often); Intensity (or how hard); Time (how long); Type (what mode or type of exercise)

So as an example, we've talked through enough benefits of exercise. You've moved into contemplation (you remember our discussion of stages of change) but the idea of the gym is intimidating and you're just not ready. We can still make a plan work. Let's commit to some simple cardiovascular exercise. You're going to walk (that's the type) for 20 minutes after dinner (that's the time) three times a week with your spouse (that's the frequency) at a gentle pace so you can talk about your day (that's the intensity). And that's great! It's a start! You're getting out the door, getting moving, and committing to improved health in a gentle way that's doable for you right now.

A month from now, you're starting to feel better, you're more energized in the morning, less stressed at work, and your pants are a little looser. So let's increase your plan. Now you're going to walk five days a week, for 30 minutes, at a little faster pace. We've increased the frequency, intensity, and time. You've also decided to add some strength and flexibility training. Twice a week you'll try the chair yoga session from the active DVDs in this course, so the frequency will be twice a week, intensity will be gentle to moderate, time will be 30 minutes, and type will be chair yoga. So now you've added something else to your fit plan.

Let's think now about what your plan is going to be. Get out your journal. Draw a table and across the top, write FITT: Frequency, Intensity, Time, and Type. Down the side, write down cardiovascular exercise, strength training, balance training, flexibility training, and pelvic floor exercise. Be deliberate; think about what you want to do, what you can really commit to right now. Start small and be realistic, because success builds to more success.

As another activity, in preparation for our next lecture, think creatively about the activity you're already doing. It may surprise you to discover that many of the things you already do may actually promote physical activity. In our next lecture, we'll talk more about different types of physical activity that can help you creatively build your physical fitness plan. By being a little bit more deliberate, you can leverage your physical activities into a bona fide exercise program!

As you work in your journal on your FITT plan, be realistic. Think about what you would enjoy, what your life will currently support, and how we can help you use the principles of FITT to start building physical fitness. What matters is that it's the plan that works for you, because this is your fitness and your healthy aging.

Fitness beyond the Gym—Active Daily Living
Lecture 5

E ven if you make good health-promoting decisions, such as getting 8 hours of sleep a night and exercising for 30 minutes 5 times a week, you still have to worry about the other 15½ hours in your day. Large-scale studies show that increased sitting raises your risk of disease and premature death, and this increased risk holds even among people who exercise regularly. The problem is that most of us sit for 12 or more hours each day. In this lecture, we'll talk about building movement into our daily lives in addition to 30 minutes a day of deliberate exercise.

The Benefits of Movement

- When you stand up and move around, your muscles contract; in turn, those muscular contractions stimulate blood flow and the movement of lymph through your body, helping to clear bacteria out of your cells. Muscle contractions also help your body clear out fats and sugars.

- Animal studies indicate that when animals rest for prolonged periods, they have decreased enzymatic activity. Most chemical reactions that occur at the cellular level require enzymatic activity; thus, decreased enzymatic activity may indicate that your body is not functioning as effectively as it should be at a cellular level.

- Thermogenesis is the production of heat by the cells of the body, in other words, the burning of calories. There are several forms of thermogenesis, including exercise-associated thermogenesis (EAT); non-exercise activity thermogenesis (NEAT); shivering thermogenesis; and diet-induced thermogenesis (DIT).
  - About 10% of food calories consumed are required to process calories in the body, and DIT is the energy required for that processing. But DIT means that all calories are not alike. A calorie of carbohydrates can take 5% to 10% of its energy just to process it; a calorie of protein can take 20% to 30% of

its energy to process; and a calorie of fat may take as little as 3% of its energy to process. Thus, a cup of full-fat ice cream not only has more calories than a cup of non-fat, high-protein Greek yogurt, but it is also easier for your body to burn, which means that you keep more of those calories.

o NEAT can be a great way to boost your metabolism and support weight loss or weight maintenance. In one research study, lean people were found to move more—up to 67% more movement in a day—and obese people were found to sit more—up to 61% more sitting in a day. In other words, fidgeting is a great way to burn calories all day long.

Activities of Daily Living
- If you get only one exercise device to support your health, it should be a pedometer. Attach it to your waistband every day and keep track of how much you walk. If you're like the average American, you will walk between 2,000 and 3,000 steps a day, but to promote health through daily movement, you should aim for 10,000 steps a day. Large-scale research studies show that middle-aged adults who accumulate more than 10,000 steps per day have more favorable body composition and a lower risk of cardiovascular disease.

- As we've said, a little goes a long way. Try to combine a little bit of exercise with a focused effort to sit less and move more. Shoot for 30 minutes a day of actual exercise, and remember that three 10-minute blocks is fine. Then, make a conscious decision to stand more than you sit and walk whenever you can.

- To incorporate more movement in your daily activities, try taking the stairs instead of the elevator, parking at the back of the parking lot, or pacing instead of sitting while on the telephone. You can also think of chores, such as raking leaves or mopping, as ways to incorporate more movement into your life. The following chart shows how many calories a 155-pound individual burns by performing some common daily activities.

Activity (performed for 30 minutes)	Calories Burned (by a 155-pound individual)
Exercise	
Walking	150
Taking a gentle yoga class	150
Taking a low-impact aerobics class	200
Riding a stationary bike	250
Running on a treadmill (at 5 miles per hour)	300
Inactivity	
Napping	23
Watching TV	27
Reading	42
Standing in line	47
Household Chores	
Raking the lawn	149
Performing general gardening	167
Weeding the garden	172
Digging and spading the garden	186
Chopping wood	223
Shoveling snow	223
Cooking	93
Working on your car	112
Grocery shopping with a cart	130
Washing windows	167
Painting the house	186
Moving furniture	223
Leisure Activities	
Playing pool or billiards	93
Going bowling or playing Frisbee	112
Practicing archery	130

Playing golf	130 (with cart)/205 (carrying clubs)
Coaching a children's sports event	149
Playing hopscotch or other active games with children	186
Ballroom or square dancing	200

- You can increase movement at work by walking to a colleague's office to talk rather than emailing, pacing while you're on the phone, or walking around the building with a colleague rather than sitting at a conference table. You might consider using a standing desk or sitting on an exercise ball rather than a standard chair.

  o Make sure your keyboard and monitor are at the right height and try to get some natural light into your work area. Research shows that people who work in office buildings that have natural or full-spectrum light have better health, reduced absenteeism, and increased productivity.

  o Be aware of your posture while you work. One research study found that when people were reminded to sit up straight, they had more confidence in their own abilities than when they were slumped over a desk.

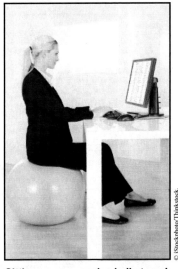

© iStockphoto/Thinkstock.

Sitting on an exercise ball at work engages your core body muscles and your back muscles, enabling you to develop your balance all day long.

Outdoor Exercise
- Japanese has a word that literally means "forest bathing"; it refers to the restorative benefits of being out in nature. Being outside can

Posture Check

If you're seated, plant your feet firmly on the floor with your and knees about hip width apart and your shoulders stacked over your hips. Roll your shoulders gently down and back, with your chest soft and open. Your head and gaze should be level, with the back of your neck neutral. Notice how you feel in this position: calm, confident, centered.

Now, as a contrast, let yourself slump forward. Drop your spine backward and let your shoulders and neck roll forward, with your head drooping downward. Feel how your body and mind become more tired. Your energy is just as "slumpy" as your posture.

Deliberately sit back up; roll your shoulders down and back and concentrate on pulling your belly button in to engage your core. Again, notice how much more stable, centered, and strong you feel.

If you really feel need to boost your energy, spread your legs wide, with your knees and hips open at angles, and feel how that "pops" your chest open and lifts you up naturally. It's actually uncomfortable to slump in a wide-legged position. When you've got a wide base, it's easier to maintain better posture.

Next, stand with your feet about hip width apart, allowing your body to stack up in alignment—ankles over feet, knees over ankles, hips over knees, shoulders over hips. Gently roll your shoulders down and back to open the chest. Your arms are relaxed beside you. Your head is neutral, and your neck is comfortable. This isn't the Marine Corps chest-popped posture; it's open, comfortable, and relaxed. Every hour throughout the day, stand up from your chair for a moment and try this deliberate stance. This exercise engages the muscles of your back and core and reduces your total sitting time during the day.

have profound health benefits, including effects on psychological health. Research indicates that walking outside can reduce depression and improve memory.

- One theory holds that nature gives our attention a break from the distractions of the modern world. When we're outdoors, we have more space to rest and allow our attention to wander, and the things that we do attend to are richly rewarding—the changing colors of leaves or the flash of a bird flying by.

- You get more benefit from a 3-mile walk on a nature trail or in a park than you do from a 3-mile walk in a mall. As you plan your exercise routine, think about taking your workout outside the gym and into the natural world. You may experience even greater benefits when fresh air, natural light, and a green landscape are combined with physical fitness activities.

Dance and Sports

- Dancing or sports allow you to experience social benefits combined with physical activity. Dancing provides aerobic exercise and is an excellent workout for improving your balance.
  - You'll find many styles of dancing to try, including ballroom dancing, line dancing, contra dancing, polka, square dancing, salsa, and Latin dancing. In addition to dance studios, you can find dance programs in community or senior citizen centers and at local community colleges or universities.

  - Learning dance routines provides mental exercise to challenge your memory and improve cognitive ability, and music can support an elevated mood. Further, the social component of dance helps you develop and strengthen relationships with others and can provide an opportunity to connect with both older and younger people.

- Even if you've never been particularly active and don't consider yourself athletic, consider trying a sport. The results may be surprising; you might find that training for a triathlon or learning tennis adds a spark of excitement to your life.

o Use the FITT plan we discussed in the last lecture to build the fitness components you need to add sports to your life. For instance, if you've always walked and would like to try running a 5-kilometer race, begin transitioning a portion of your walking time to running. Try walking for 15 minutes, running for 5, and walking for 15 more minutes. When you begin to feel comfortable with that routine, add more running time.

o Before you get started with a new sport, talk to your doctor to make you understand any safety recommendations you should follow. For instance, if you've had a knee replacement or have a history of stress fractures in your feet, running may not be the right goal for you to set.

o You may also consider making an investment in the process. Hire an instructor or coach to learn correct form and strategies, which will help you stay safe. And make sure you have appropriate equipment.

Exercise on Vacation
- Think about your vacation as another opportunity to get moving. A vacation doesn't have to mean that you just pay money and eat food. Even on a cruise ship, you'll find numerous opportunities for activity. Many ships have rock walls to climb or surfing machines, dance or fitness classes, and personal trainers. Without your work schedule and the stressors of daily life to get in your way, you can spend time taking better care of your body.

- Of course, on vacation, you can also go exploring. On a cruise, instead of signing up for a bus tour in port, try swimming with stingrays or zip-lining across the rain forest. Think about opportunities for eustress and surprise yourself with activities that are fun, different, interesting.

- Consider planning your whole vacation around physical activities. If you love to bike, plan a biking tour of French wine country. If you're into hiking, try a volksmarching tour in Germany. Build fitness into the planning stages of your vacation to heighten your sense of anticipation and the fun once you arrive at your destination.

Suggested Reading

Buder, *The Grace to Race.*

Levine, *Move a Little, Lose a Lot.*

National Senior Games Association, www.nsga.com.

Switzer, *Running and Walking for Women over 40.*

Team Hoyt, www.teamhoyt.com.

Activities and Assignments

Go back to the list of activities to leverage as creative approaches to exercise that you generated in Lecture 4. Assess how many of them qualify as activity based on calories burned. Which ones burn as many calories as a 30-minute workout? How can you turn those activities into workouts? For instance, do you do enough yard work for a dedicated 10-, 20-, or 30-minute block of active gardening? Visit http://www.health.harvard.edu/newsweek/Calories-burned-in-30-minutes-of-leisure-and-routine-activities.htm for a list of calories burned by various activities for individuals weighing 125 pounds, 155 pounds, and 185 pounds.

How can you stretch yourself to try something new? What's a fitness activity you have always wanted to try but haven't thought you could do? How can you challenge your preconceived notions and surprise yourself? Think about the practical components—equipment, instruction, and location—so that you can use logistical planning to set yourself up for success.

Fitness beyond the Gym—Active Daily Living
Lecture 5—Transcript

Here's something you can put in the "not fair" category: Even if you make good health-promoting decisions like getting eight hours of sleep a night, and exercising for 30 minutes every day, you still have to worry about the other 15.5 hours in your day. Large-scale studies show that increased sitting raises your risk of disease and premature death. This increased risk holds even among people who exercise regularly.

Researchers in one large study found that sitting was a risk factor for illness and death even after they controlled for age, gender, smoking status, physical activity, education, body mass index, and whether the individual lived in an urban or rural environment. People who sat for more than 11 hours a day were at the greatest risk, with those who sat for less than 4 hours per day at the lowest risk.

Think about it. You sit at the table for every meal. You sit in your car for at least 50 minutes a day, since the U.S. Census says the average work commute is 25 minutes each direction. In the current workforce, most of us have jobs that require us to sit at desks working on computers, so we sit at our desks for 8 or 10 or 12 hours a day while we work. Then maybe, at night, to relax a little, we sit on our couches and watch some television. In fact, we spend 90 percent of our leisure time sitting down. All of that sitting adds up to lot of time that our muscles aren't moving.

When you stand and move, your muscles contract, and those muscular contractions stimulate blood flow and the movement of lymph through your body. Lymph is important because the lymphatic system is closely related to the immune system, and the lymph nodes help the body clear bacteria out of your cells. Muscle contractions also help your body clear fats and sugars from your body. Animal studies indicate that when animals rest for prolonged periods, they have decreased enzymatic activity. Most chemical reactions that occur at the cellular level require enzymatic activity, so decreased enzymatic activity may indicate that your body is not functioning as effectively as it should, at a cellular level.

Thermogenesis is the production of heat by the cells of the body—in other words, the burning of calories. There are several forms of thermogenesis; for instance, exercise-associated thermogenesis, or EAT; non-exercise activity thermogenesis, or NEAT; shivering thermogenesis, which is the amount of calories your body burns trying to stay warm; and diet-induced thermogenesis, or DIT. Diet-induced thermogenesis is the energy required to process your food; about 10 percent of food calories consumed are required to process them in the body. Interestingly, diet-induced thermogenesis means that a calorie is not a calorie. A calorie of carbohydrates can take 5–10 percent of its energy just to process it. A calorie of protein can take 20–30 percent of its energy to process it, and a calorie of fat may take as little as 3 percent of its energy to process it. So a cup of full-fat ice cream not only has more calories than a cup of non-fat, high-protein Greek yogurt, it also is easier for your body to retain those calories from the full-fat ice cream. You keep more of those calories.

NEAT, or non-exercise activity thermogenesis, can be a great way to boost your metabolism and support weight loss or weight maintenance. In one research study, lean individuals were compared to obese individuals. Participants were asked to wear undergarments that were studded with sensors that tracked movement. The study found that the lean people moved more, up to 67 percent more movement in a day, and the obese people sat more, up to 61 percent more sitting in a day.

When I first read that study years ago, I actually called my mother to tell her she was wrong when she always told me as a kid to sit still and stop fidgeting. Fidgeting, as it turns it out, is a great way to burn calories all day long. So pace your office while you talk on the phone, stretch your hands and feet while you work at your desk, and find as many ways as you can to move in little ways throughout your day. For the sake of your office mates, family, and friends, don't take it too far. I'm not telling you to click your pen all day long or snap your gum and try to justify it as NEAT.

In this lecture, we'll focus on fitness outside the gym. So let's start by talking about activities of daily living, all of the ways that we can get off our bottoms and build movement into our daily lives. Your 30 minutes of exercise a day is important for a whole lot of health reasons. But so are the small decisions you make throughout the other 15.5 hours of your waking day.

If you only get one exercise devise to support your health, it should be a pedometer. Attach it to your waistband every day, and keep track of how much you're walking. If you're like the average American, you will walk between 2,000 and 3,000 steps a day. This is connected back to the fact that we all sit too darn much. To promote your health through daily movement, you should aim for 10,000 steps a day. Large-scale research studies show that middle-aged adults who accumulate more than 10,000 steps per day have a more favorable body composition, and a lower risk of cardiovascular disease.

This is a place where an old-fashioned lifestyle may pay off. A study of Amish men and women found that the average Amish man takes more than 18,000 steps per day, and the average Amish woman takes more than 14,000 steps per day. They don't have gym memberships, they don't use free weights, and they don't plan exercise programs. But they are active: Amish men perform 65 hours of activity a week, and Amish women perform 48 hours of activity a week. When you make some comparisons, among Americans, 69 percent are overweight and 36 percent are obese. When you look at the Amish, though, only 26 percent are overweight and only 4 percent are obese, in spite of the fact that a traditional Amish diet is very high calorie and has a high fat content.

So it bears repeating: A little goes a long way, especially if you combine a little bit of exercise with a focused effort to sit less and move more. Shoot for 30 minutes a day of actual exercise, and remember that three 10-minute blocks are fine. Then, make a conscious decision to stand more than you sit, and walk whenever you can. Think about how to make deliberate decision. Take the stairs instead of the elevator, park at the back of the parking lot, pace while you're on the telephone instead of just sitting there. Engage in the kinds of activities of daily living that can actually promote physical fitness. Think of things like manual household work, chores in your yard, raking leaves, mowing with a lawnmower manually instead of riding it, sweeping, mopping, dusting. These all require bending, reaching, and physical exertion.

Let's set some context for a minute. We'll look through the amount of calories an average, 155-pound person would burn in a couple of different exercise scenarios, doing 30 minutes of activity each time. That 155-pound person would burn on a 30-minute walk about 150 calories. Same 150 calories if they took a 30-minute gentle yoga class. Low-impact aerobics class, 30 minutes—200 calories. Riding a stationary bike for 30 minutes: 250 calories. Running 5 miles per hour for 30 minutes on the treadmill: 300 calories.

That same 155-pound person during the non-active periods of the day: If they were sleeping 30 minutes, they would burn 23 calories. If they were watching TV for 30 minutes, only 27 calories. Sitting and reading for 30 minutes: 42 calories. Standing in line for 30 minutes: 47 calories. So you'll notice, if you're reading, which requires mental energy, or standing, which requires some physical effort, you'll burn twice as many calories as sleeping or sitting and watching TV. You can also get a nice calorie burn by making choices about the rest of your day, by choosing to do activities in your home and leisure time that burn calories and promote fitness. Let's take a look at a few more examples of how many calories that same 155-pound person would burn in 30 minutes of activities around the house.

For instance, if you go out to the yard, do some yardwork for 30 minutes? Raking the lawn: 149 calories. General gardening: 167 calories. Weeding the garden: 172 calories. Digging and spading in the garden: 186 calories. Chopping wood: 223; shoveling snow: 223. More things that you can do around your house. Actually, cooking: 93 calories. Working on your car: 112. Grocery shopping, when you're pushing a cart: 130 calories. Washing windows: 167. Thirty minutes of washing windows and you've done more than if you went for a half-hour walk or took a half-hour yoga class. Painting the house: 186 calories. Moving furniture: 223 calories.

And what about your leisure time? How could you use that time instead of just watching TV for 30 minutes? Maybe you go out and play pool or billiards. In 30 minutes you're going to burn 93 calories. You could go bowling, play Frisbee: 112 calories in calories in 30 minutes. Playing archery: 130 calories in 30 minutes. Golf: If you're using a cart, it's 130 calories for 30 minutes, but if you're carrying your own clubs, 205 calories.

So if you carried your clubs over two hours on the back nine holes, you'd burn over 800 calories. Any time you get into a "is golf a sport or is golf not a sport debate," think about playing while carrying your own clubs, and it really becomes an active sport.

You can even do some activities with your kids or spouse. If you coach at your kid's sports event, moving around with the kids, 149 calories in 30 minutes. Get a little more active, play hopscotch, jump rope, some sort of active game: 186 calories in 30 minutes. Or go out dancing with your spouse: 200 calories in 30 minutes. Go out for an hour, dance with your spouse, you've burned more calories than if you went for a two-mile run.

Let's think about work now, because if you're doing the right thing , you're sleeping eight hours a night, you're spending 33 percent of your time in sleep. You work another 40–60 hours a week, you're spending another third of your week at work. So the decisions you make in your workplace can have a profound impact on your health. That's why it's important that you think about how you structure your office environment; how do you set yourself up for success to promote your health. You want to make sure that your office environment does not abuse or damage your health. You also want to make sure that it does not compromise your motivation to do health-promoting activities.

There are small simple choices you can make to move more while you're at work. For instance, think about, can you walk across the hall to talk with a colleague, rather than just emailing someone who works in the same office? You might even have a better conversation face-to-face rather than getting caught in the nuances of email. You can get up while you're on the phone and pace around, rather than sitting at your desk. If you're sitting at your desk and you're typing or working, get up every hour and stretch, so that you're not sitting for too long. Even five minutes every hour is going to help with that movement of your body, activating your muscles. Think about, rather than sitting around a conference table to brainstorm, you can go out for a walk with your colleagues and brainstorm. You might even find you have better ideas by getting outside into a different environment into some open space.

Think about being sneaky with yourself. Don't make life so easy. Put your trashcan and your office supplies on the opposite side of your office from your desk. Every time you throw something away or need a new pen, you actually have to get up and walk across your office.

You can also make furniture choices to support your fitness. For instance, have you ever seen a standing desk? You probably have at your doctor's office. They often have them for the doctor to quickly take notes in the patient room. Think about, would that be helpful in your office so that you could stand up more? You could even try a desk over a treadmill. It sounds unusual, but some advocates of NEAT—non-exercise activity thermogenesis—support the idea of walking at a very slow pace, just 1–2 miles per hour, while you work. It may take a few weeks to readjust how you work your mouse and your keyboard, but you may find it very helpful in getting you up and moving.

You can also try sitting on an exercise ball. Some of them have sand in the bottom so they don't roll around; others come with bases and backs to make them a little more like desk chairs, give you a little bit more stability. But whatever the form, those bouncy-ball chairs engage your core body muscles and back muscles so that you can work on your balance all day long.

I have exercise balls for my office desk chairs, and we have them around our kitchen table instead of kitchen chairs. I even have little tiny ones for my children. There's some research studies that schools have found that for children with hyperactivity issues, sitting on a balance ball chair can provide small amounts of movement, focused fidgeting if you will, to help them stay more on task during the school day.

Think about other ergonomic decisions as well, though, like the right height for your keyboard, the right height for your computer monitor, having natural light, being able to see outside, because how your office is set up can have profound impacts on your physical and psychological health. For instance, natural light: Research shows that people who work in office buildings that have natural light or full-spectrum light have better health, reduced absenteeism, and increased productivity. Headaches and eyestrain, in particular, can be related to insufficient light levels. Some European countries actually regulate that workers must be within 27 feet of a window, because of the benefits of natural light. Natural light is best, but full-spectrum bright lights can be an effective option when natural light isn't possible. The health impacts can be particularly pronounced for individuals with Seasonal Affective Disorder, but they have a benefit for everyone.

When individuals have windows with the capacity to look out on a long-range view, it can actually reduce eyestrain by providing an opportunity to refocus your gaze. So as you work at your computer and you're looking very close, be deliberate, make time to look away. Look out the window. Ideally, you'd be looking out a window at a natural setting as well, because research has found that looking at green, natural spaces can actually improve your attention and reduce blood pressure. If you're in a windowless office, then have some green plants around to help provide a similar stress-reducing benefit.

Let's talk about posture for a moment. One research study found that when people were reminded to sit up straight, they had more confidence in their own abilities than when they were slumped over a desk. So while the old adage that standing up straight makes you look better holds true, it also appears that standing up straight actually makes you feel better. So, if you're at work and you're feeling tired or unsure or worn down, stop and do a physical body check. Let's grab a chair and try this.

Here's one of the bouncy-ball chairs I was just talking about. We'll use it for our posture check. If you're seated, come into a comfortable position with your feet and knees about hip-width apart. Yes, it's more ladylike to keep your knees together, or to cross your ankles: It's a great reason to wear pants, you can work better on your posture. Your feet are planted firmly on the floor, providing a good foundation. Nice, comfortable stacked spine, shoulders are stacked over hips, rolled gently down and back, chest soft and open. The back of the neck is neutral, the head is level, your gaze is even and level. Overall it's a very nice, comfortable, open posture.

Do a body check. See how you feel while sitting like this: calm, confident, centered. Grounded in your body. Try a contrast to that; let yourself shlump forward. Drop your spine backward, let your shoulders roll forward. You're sitting at your desk; you've been here all day long. Your neck is rolled forward, your head is unlevel. Feel how your body and mind are actually more tired. Your energy becomes as shlumpy as your posture.

Again, contrast that. Deliberately sit back up, roll the shoulders down and back, concentrate on pulling your belly button in to engage your core; feel how much more stable and centered, and strong you're feeling.

If you really feel like you need to boost your energy and get up some internal power, spread your legs wide, your knees and hips open up at angles, and feel how that "pops" your chest open and lifts you up naturally. It's very hard to shlump in a wide-legged position. Try it for a moment, and feel how uncomfortable that is on your low back. When you've got a wide base, it's easier to maintain better posture, so if you're thinking deliberately about your posture, working on your posture, it can be a good exercise to sit wide-legged for a while, helping you to promote that posture while you build up the core-body strength and the muscles of your back and abdominal muscles.

Now, let's do the same posture check while standing.

Come on up to standing, and your feet are about hip-width apart, allow your body to stack: ankles over feet, knees over ankles, hips over knees, shoulders over hips. Gently, roll your shoulders down and back to open the chest. Your arms are relaxed beside you. Your head is neutral, your neck is comfortable. We're not doing a Marine Corps posture where your chest is popped open. We're just comfortable, relaxed, tall.

Throughout the day, stand up from your chair for a moment, and be deliberate about your posture. It's great exercise; it engages the muscles of your back and your core. For women in particular, it's a great way to stay strong and open in the chest and prevent the dowager's hump that can start to happen with age. It will get harder as you get older—osteoporosis and spine degeneration make it harder to stand up straight and keep good posture, which makes it all the more important that you practice regularly and build up your muscle strength so that you can maintain good posture. And again, if you stand up every hour and work on your posture for a few minutes, it will help build muscular strength and reduce your total sitting time.

In Japanese, they have a word which literally means "Forest Bathing" and it refers to the restorative benefits of being out in nature. Being outside can have profound health benefits: clean air, lack of noise pollution; some studies even suggest benefits from wood essential oils. Outdoor activity can also have profound effects on our psychological health, with research studies indicating that walking outside can actually reduce depression and improve memory. One theory proposes that nature gives our attention a break. In particular, in the modern world there are so many things competing for our attention: traffic lights, ringing cell phones, the people around us. We're forced to pay attention throughout the day to stay safe and on task. In contrast, in nature, we have more space to rest and allow our attention to wander, but at the same time, as our mind wanders, our involuntary attention is actually richly rewarded with detail, color, the sounds of nature. We're walking along and we notice the color of a blade of grass, the color of the changing leaves, a bird that flashes by, a squirrel in your peripheral vision.

So what this all boils down to as practical guidance is that you get more benefit from a three-mile walk on a nature trail or in a park than you do from a three-mile walk around a mall. An outdoor track would provide some of the outdoor benefits, particularly if it was in an open, green space and you were outside. So as you plan your exercise routine, think about how you can take your workout out of the gym and into the natural world. You may experience improved benefits when you've got fresh air, natural light, and a green landscape combined with your physical fitness activities.

You can also bring together social benefits with your physical activity if you try something like dancing. Dancing provides an aerobic exercise which is an excellent workout that also improves your balance. There are many styles to try: ballroom dancing, line dancing, contra dancing, polka, square dancing, salsa, Latin dancing, you could even try the hustle, which is always to fun, upbeat 70s-era music. There are styles of dancing that work both with or without a partner, so it doesn't matter if you have someone to go with or you're going to try it alone. And there are many places to get started—dance studios of course, but most communities also have dance classes and dance programs in community centers, senior citizen community centers, local university continuing-education programs, or lodges like a Mason lodge or a VFW.

Learning dance routines also provides mental exercise to challenge your memory and improve cognitive ability as you're learning and memorizing patterns. Music has also been found to support elevated mood. Further, that social component of dance is great for helping you develop and strengthen relationships with others. It can also be a fun intergenerational opportunity, to connect people both older and younger than you are. You may be surprised at those dancing across the age spectrum, especially at community dances. You may remember my friend Joe who we talked about in Lecture 2, when we discussed motivation; in his 80s, Joe was attending the university dance club and helping teach young women, high-school and college age, how to dance.

Dance can even keep people connected in the most challenging circumstances. Years ago, I knew a couple who had been dance teachers when they were younger. The wife had late-stage Alzheimer's and had to live in a care facility, because her husband couldn't take care of her by himself anymore. But every Tuesday afternoon, he'd pick her up and he'd take her to the local VFW for a swing dance where there was a live big band playing swing-dance music. Even though she still didn't remember his name, they danced just as they always had, and she remembered how to do every step, every turn, and for a few hours each week, he felt like he got his wife back and they connected with each other, the way they'd connected throughout their whole life.

Another thing to think about, even if you haven't been particularly active, even if you don't consider yourself athletic, consider trying a sport. You might surprise yourself. You might find that training for a triathlon or learning tennis or joining a volleyball team adds a new spark of excitement to your life.

If you want to try a sport, be deliberate, make a plan. When we get to Lecture 7, motivation part 2, we'll talk about SMART goals; you can use SMART goals to build a path to the sports outcome you want. You will also use the FITT plan that we discussed in our lecture on fitness fundamentals so that you can build the fitness components you need to get started. For instance, if you've always walked, maybe you want to move up to running and you want to try a five-kilometer race, think about how to build a plan for that.

How much, how fast, and how often do you walk now? That's where you're starting. You're going to start by transitioning a portion of your walk time to running. Maybe you start out walking 15 minutes to warm up, then you run for 5 minutes, and then you walk for 15 more minutes to cool down and relax. It's a small step, but it's realistic, it's doable, there's a low likelihood of you getting injured, so it gives you an initial success from which you can move forward. As you feel more comfortable, as you make it to 5 minutes of running without losing your breath and getting a side stitch, you add more time. Eventually you work up to a full 30 minutes of running. Once that feels good, you work up to 5 kilometers. Once you successfully complete 5 kilometers, you set your sights on your next goal, and you build a plan towards that.

For instance, perhaps you want to work up to a 10-kilometer run, and eventually a marathon. Even if you know the marathon is your eventual goal, you should still start with the 5K because success leads to success, and small successes are easier to work toward and achieve. Think about the mental strategies you need; for instance, try using the mindfulness strategies we will discuss in our next lecture to keep you focused and help you work through challenges. If you wake up tired and achy after your first few runs, how will you talk yourself through it that so you can keep going?

If you're going to try sports for the first time, before you get started, consider your own health and talk to your doctor, make you understand any safety recommendations which you should follow based on your health. If you've had a knee replacement or have a history of stress fractures in your feet, running might not be the right goal for you to set. Maybe you try training to compete as a swimmer. Something that has less likelihood of hurting your knees and your feet. Think about your body.

You will want to invest in the process. Hire an instructor to learn the right form, the right strategies, to keep you safe. Also make sure you have the appropriate equipment; if you're trying to run, you need the right shoes: You shouldn't just head out in your walking shoes. You should also look for any needed safety gear, based on the activity. Because you are older, if you get hurt, it will take longer for you to heal. You have less margin for error, and because of that, you need to be more careful where it counts.

But don't be discouraged by your possibly false beliefs. Just because you haven't considered it before or done it before, doesn't mean you can't do it. Just because it seems like something only other people do, doesn't mean you shouldn't try. Get real information based on your health history and your interests, and set appropriate goals from there to challenge yourself and try something new.

Also challenge yourself to think about vacation as another opportunity to move. Vacation doesn't just have to mean that you pay money and eat food. Think about a cruise ship, the classic place where people stuff themselves from the opulent buffets; think of all the opportunities for activity instead. On the new big ships, you could try out activities like rock-wall climbing, surfing. Most ships have personal trainers, and without your work schedule and the stressors of daily life in your way, you could do some much-needed self-care, and learn how to take better care of your body.

On a ship, you can hike and explore in the ports of call. You can take the stairs and check out the hidden gems of artwork on every floor, instead of waiting in line for the elevator you can be exploring the whole shit. You could try a dance class, even seek out one of those dance-focused cruises. Instead of taking a party boat, when you get into port you could try swimming with the stingrays or zip lining across the rain forest. Surprise yourself with something fun, something different, something interesting. Think about opportunities for eustress; be safe, but challenge yourself to have fun with some calculated risks.

Think also about interesting different places that you could do exercise in settings you've never explored when you're thinking about vacations. Maybe you love to bike. What about if you took a wine-and-bike tour across the French countryside? Maybe you've always wanted to try kayaking; you could try evening kayaking in Puerto Rico in one of the bioluminescent bays, where every time your oar moves through the water, it bumps these little microorganisms that then sparkle like fireflies, the water glows in the dark. Maybe you love to hike. You could head to Germany and try a volksmarching tour of Germany where you'll get a walking stick and you'll get a metal flag every time you finish a walk as a memento to take home for your walks across Germany. And then, you can use your preparation and planning to build fitness in early, creating a sense of anticipation and excitement. You're going to go on that bike tour across France, you start biking at home, logging in miles as you save up money towards the trip. Or you are gonna kayak in Puerto Rico, so you learn how to kayak in a local lake, discovering how it feels, how much it challenges your legs, learning all about the way to kayak and maintain your balance in the water. If you're counting down to your flight to Germany you hike in different parks in your neighborhood, so that you're preparing yourself for your adventure.

For this lecture's takeaway activities, I'd like you to look at both ends of the spectrum. First, let's look at your daily routine. At the end of Lecture 4, I asked you to brainstorm what activities you're already doing that you could leverage as creative approaches to exercise. For one takeaway activity today, go back to that list and assess how many of them would qualify as activity based on calories burned. Which ones are burning as many calories as a 30-minute workout? How can you then turn those activities into workouts? For instance, do you do enough yardwork to do at least a dedicated 10- or 20- or 30-minute block of active gardening?

Then, let's look at the rainbow. What have you always wanted to try? How can you stretch yourself to try something new? What's a fitness activity you have always wanted to try, but haven't thought you could do it? How can you challenge your preconceived notions about who you are and what your ability is? How can you surprise yourself? Once you've identified that fitness dream, think about how can you set yourself up to give it a go. Focus on practical components, equipment, instruction, and location, so that you can use logistical planning to eliminate your excuses and give you the psychological energy to try it. What's the worst that could happen? What's the best outcome that you could achieve?

Exercise means deliberate fitness programs, such as a class at the gym or a weightlifting routine. However, you can stay fit and healthy without ever stepping foot in the gym. What you need is a conscious intent to be physically fit, so that you engage regularly in physical activities. A broad array of activities can support physical fitness, and you can try activities like sports or dance classes. In our next lecture, we'll discuss mindful fitness strategies such as yoga and tai chi, and how they can be an important part of your overall fitness program. You can also build your fitness through activities of daily living. In fact, I'd encourage you to focus in particular on your activities of daily living, and figure out how to build more movement in throughout your day. Because in the end, the gym membership doesn't matter. What matters is that you sit less and move more.

It's Not Just Physical—Mindful Fitness
Lecture 6

W e've spent the last few lectures talking about things you can do to improve your health, such as getting more sleep, eating a healthy diet, and of course, exercising. But when we talk about fitness, it's important to think holistically. All those health-promoting practices are components of a larger picture. We are more than our bodies, and health is more than just good food and regular exercise. Along with the physical, we need to consider the cognitive, psychological, social, and spiritual components of our lives. In this lecture, we will focus on mindfulness fitness practices—types of exercise intended to help you feel the sense of unity between your mind and body.

An Introduction to Mindful Fitness

- Mindful fitness practices use a combination of physical and psychological exercise to cultivate both physical and psychological health and wellness. These programs include yoga, Tai Chi, and the martial arts, all of which combine physical exercise with deliberate breathing and mental training.

- Mindful fitness practices provide physical fitness benefits, such as strength, flexibility, and balance training, but they also offer benefits beyond physical exercise. The research literature shows that mindfulness practices are particularly well suited to supporting mental health and well-being, improving self-esteem, reducing depression and anxiety, and even reducing perceptions of pain. Mindfulness practices may be particularly appropriate for older adults, because they offer gentle, well-rounded fitness programs with a focus on balance and overall strength and a low risk for injury.

- Mindfulness practices are part of the broad spectrum of holistic approaches to health known as complementary and alternative medicine (CAM). One cross-sectional study found that 63% of older adults had used at least one CAM modality, with an average of three CAM approaches per person. Many people use CAM therapies to support their health and wellness: 34% reported using CAM for anxiety; 27%, for depression; 19%, for chronic pain; 18%, for heart diseases; 13%, for insomnia; and 12%, for fatigue.

- Because they are inherently gentle, these low-risk exercise programs are appropriate for older adults. There is also some benefit to coming to mindfulness practices when you are older and bring with you a desire to be more introspective.

- Mindful fitness programs offer a low-threat way to promote health. As a culture, we may be uncomfortable talking about stress or anxiety, but we can go to a yoga class without stigma and learn breathing and focusing techniques that help us deal with these issues. Mindful practices also support our sense of being self-sufficient and independent; they allow us to feel in control of our own care and well-being.

- Some people may be hesitant about mindful fitness because of their own religious or philosophical beliefs, but mindfulness practices can actually enhance your spirituality, allowing you to be more present—more fully in the moment—during your religious practice.

- Not all mindfulness classes are suited to everyone; different instructors have different approaches to teaching these practices. Feel free to try out various classes to find the approach and the instructor that make you most comfortable.

Yoga

- The Sanskrit word *yoga* means "union." Yoga brings together physical and psychological exercise to cultivate both physical and psychological health and wellness. It is an exercise practice that is built on a cohesive philosophy and is now supported by solid empirical research. You could do psychological skills training and physical exercise as separate and isolated components, but with yoga, you have the opportunity to train both aspects of yourself in an integrated way.

- Although yoga has its background and history in the Indian tradition and the Hindu religion, yoga itself is a pragmatic and adaptable practice. At its core, yoga is a practice intended to bring about unity of the mind and body. Through physical exercise, focused attention, and deliberate breathing, you can enhance the sense of connection between your internal and external self.

- Yoga is uniquely effective in helping you manage and cope with stress. Over time, a consistent yoga practice reduces your reactivity to stress, both physiologically and psychologically. The common ways we physically manifest stress—rapid breathing, elevated heart rate, and muscular tension—are all improved through regular yoga practice. Yoga also provides a set of tools that you can use in response to stressful situations. When you practice yoga, you learn self-soothing skills that you can rely on as needed in stressful situations.

- These two stress-reducing effects of yoga practice can lead to powerful outcomes. Magnetic resonance imaging (MRI) studies show that practicing yoga can change the structure of the brain, in particular, the amygdala, a part of the brain associated with stress. Yoga practice can also change your hormone profile and how your body processes the physiological effects of stress; improve lung function; reduce symptoms of allergies; and positively affect blood-glucose levels, cholesterol levels, and overall cardiovascular risk profile.

Tai Chi and Qigong

- Tai Chi and Qigong are traditional forms of mindful exercise from China. *Qi* is the Chinese word for "energy" or "life force," and Chinese traditional medicine believes that *qi* flows through energy pathways in the body called meridians. Blocked or unbalanced *qi* can lead to illness or injury. The practices of Tai Chi and Qigong

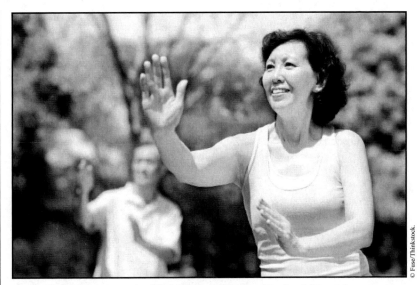
The deliberate movements of Tai Chi are often practiced outside and can resemble beautiful choreography.

are intended to support healthy energy flow and, thus, to promote overall health and well-being.

- Also foundational to the philosophy of Tai Chi and Qigong is the idea of yin and yang, or opposites. The philosophical belief is that nature consists of opposing forces—yin and yang—in appropriate balance. Tai Chi and Qigong provide balanced yet opposite movements (open and closed, hard and soft) to support the appropriate equilibrium of yin and yang in the body.

- Tai Chi and Qigong are distinct practices but are often practiced together. Tai Chi uses a specific series of movements, done as a meditation, to move *qi* in the body. Qigong includes many different exercises that may be done in different sequences and is often considered a foundational exercise before individuals begin practicing the Tai Chi sequence. Movement is never forced and muscles stay relaxed. The joints are neither fully extended nor fully

Karate Punch

Assume a wide stance, with your feet apart and firmly planted and your knees gently bent. Your legs should feel strong and solid, connecting you to the earth. Make fists with your hands, curling your fingers in and closing your thumbs on top, rather than tucked inside. Your shoulders should be rolled down and back, with your elbows bent and arms gently at your side.

Take a deep inhalation and punch your right arm out—straight and strong—with a sharp, loud exhalation through the mouth. That strong exhalation is called the *kiai*, and it literally means "shout" or "spirit" in Japanese. It adds force and power to your movement.

Take five punches on each side. Punch strong and follow through, keeping your squat steady and your posture solid. Return the opposite arm in toward your side, almost as if you are protecting your side. Exhale as you bring your arms down to your sides, then step your feet back together.

bent, and the connective tissues are not stretched. The exercises can be adapted to any fitness level.

• The movements of Tai Chi and Qigong are different from other forms of exercise because they are usually circular, as if the practitioner is moving through water. Tai Chi has often been called meditation in motion because it is a form of meditative practice, of focusing the mind and awareness through movement.

• Both Tai Chi and Qigong are beneficial for helping to maintain or improve posture and balance. These exercises are gentle on the joints and helpful in managing chronic pain and maintaining flexibility. Tai Chi and Qigong also improve strength, may promote bone density, reduce the risk for heart disease and lower blood pressure by reducing stress, and promote quality and duration of sleep. Both practices may be beneficial for those recovering from a stroke or individuals who have Parkinson's disease or arthritis.

Martial Arts

- A systematic research review conducted by the Department of Sports Medicine at Chengdu Sport University in China found that martial arts may promote health and wellness and that more research studies are warranted to validate those effects.

- Practicing martial arts gives you a wonderful opportunity to find your inner strength, especially if you are going through a tough time in life or have always been quiet and introverted. Above all, the martial arts emphasize internal control, focus, and deliberate awareness. The practice of martial arts is truly an active, moving meditation.

- Again, it's important to find the right instructor for your learning style, age, and health. Some instructors require sparring, while others allow you to learn the *katas*, which are patterns or forms of movement, without having to make contact with others.

Meditation

- Meditation is focused awareness, the deliberate training of the mind to reduce the ongoing jumble of thoughts that we live with most of the time. Meditation is always a part of mindfulness fitness practices, and if you attend a yoga, Tai Chi, or martial arts class, you will spend some time practicing meditation. You can also practice meditation on its own.

- According to the renowned meditation teacher Jack Kornfield, the mind is like a puppy you are trying to house train; you put down paper, and the puppy wanders off and goes to the bathroom in the corner. But you continue to pick the puppy up gently and bring it back to the paper. The mind is similar; you focus your awareness, but your mind wanders off somewhere else. Gently, you bring it back. Through that process—the gentle but consistent retuning to deliberate focus—you can learn to control your mind and your thoughts.

- Learning control of your mind has powerful outcomes. Psychologically, meditation helps you gain perspective, manage stress, increase your sense of self-awareness, learn to focus on the present, and reduce negative emotions. It can also have profound impacts on physical health. Research suggests that meditation can help with allergies, asthma, heart disease and high blood pressure, and even cancer, as well as conditions that involve a sense of self-control, such as binge eating or substance abuse.

- As we age, we often begin to feel a divergence between a mind that remains young and a body that is beginning to show some effects of age. Both meditation and mindfulness practices can help us stay connected to our bodies and compassionately accept the changes we experience with age.

Suggested Reading

Center for Mindfulness, http://www.umassmed.edu/content.aspx?id=41254.

Kabat-Zinn, *Mindfulness for Beginners*.

Kornfield, *The Inner Art of Meditation* (audio CD).

————, http://www.jackkornfield.com.

Muesse, *Practicing Mindfulness*.

Activities and Assignments

Sit down by yourself in a quiet space with your journal and a pen. Set a timer for 15 minutes and let your mind wander. Don't try to think of anything in particular or focus on a certain topic. Jot down a few key words for each thought you have. Don't judge your thoughts, and don't try to direct them anywhere in particular; just become aware of them and record them as they come. Write down a few words to capture the stream of consciousness. When you're done, read over what you've written. Your thoughts likely jumped around quickly from topic to topic—a task to complete at work, a fight with your spouse, something you need to buy at the grocery store, the windows that need to be cleaned, where you want to go on your vacation this year. The point of the exercise is to be aware of how much our minds move.

Pick a day and set a timer on your phone, your computer, or your watch to go off every hour during the day. In your journal, make a chart with four columns like the one shown below. Whenever your alarm goes off, write down one sentence to indicate what you're thinking about in the appropriate column—past, present, or future. Again, don't judge or try to direct your thoughts; just be aware of them and jot them down. At the end of the day, look at the overall picture and assess how much time you spent in the past, how much time you spent in the future, and probably how little time you spent in the present.

Time of Day	Past	Present	Future
7 a.m.			
8 a.m.			
9 a.m.			
...			

It's Not Just Physical—Mindful Fitness
Lecture 6—Transcript

We spent the last few lectures talking about things that you can do to improve your health. You can get more sleep, eat a healthy diet, manage your stress, and exercise. I'd like you to look at all of those health-promoting practices as important components of a larger picture. Think, for a second, if you have a friend who is in great physical shape and looks attractive, but who doesn't actually have a healthy life or a healthy sense of self.

It's important when we talk about fitness that we think holistically. We are more than our bodies, and health is more than just good food and regular exercise. We also need to nurture our internal lives, our sense of self, our sense of who we are and where we belong. Along with the physical, we need to consider the cognitive, psychological, social, and spiritual components of our lives. This can help us feel better about ourselves as we age, and embrace aging as a positive experience.

You're never quite so aware of your body until it starts to fail you. You wake up, you've had a good night's sleep, you don't recall doing anything, but you can't turn your head or your lower back is locked in place. Or you go to open a jar, and you just can't do it. Or you stay out late with friends, and you feel wrecked the next day. Inside, you still feel 25 or 30 or 40, but your body has other ideas. It's important to healthy aging to realize that you are more than just your body. It's vital to realize that for whatever physical obstacles you will experience through aging, there are other benefits: an understanding of things that used to bewilder you, a sense of acceptance for things that used to make you afraid, a sense of self-confidence built by a lifetime of success.

In this lecture, we will focus on mindfulness fitness practices, which are types of exercises intended to help you feel the sense of unity between your mind and body. They focus on helping you connect to the connection that is already there between your physical self, and your psychological self. Mindfulness practices use a combination of physical and psychological exercise to cultivate both physical and psychological health and wellness. Mindful fitness practices include programs like yoga, tai chi, and the martial arts, which combine physical exercise with deliberate breathing and mental-skills training.

Mindful fitness practices provide physical benefits for your health, such as strength, flexibility, and balance training, but they also offer benefits beyond physical exercise. The research literature shows that mindfulness practices are particularly well suited to supporting mental health and well-being, helping improve self-esteem, reducing depression and anxiety, and even reducing perceptions of pain. For instance, when pain feels unbearable, that is often related to our fear of it never ending. When we can come back to the present moment and manage just this moment, we are better able to withstand pain. We'll talk more about pain in Lecture 10, which focuses on chronic illnesses, including chronic pain. You can also try the Reiki active session, which offers a brief exercise in focusing on your body in the present moment.

Mindfulness practices may be particularly well suited for older adults, as they offer gentle, well-rounded fitness programs with a focus on balance and overall strength, with a low risk for injury. If you try mindfulness practices, which are part of the broad spectrum of holistic approaches to health known as Complementary and Alternative Medicine, or CAM, you are not alone. One cross-sectional study found that 63 percent of older adults had used at least one CAM modality, with an average of three CAM approaches per person. Many people are using CAM therapies to support their health and wellness: 34 percent reported using CAM for anxiety, 27 percent for depression, 19 percent for chronic pain, 18 percent for heart diseases, 13 percent for insomnia, and 12 percent for fatigue. For yoga in particular, 64 percent of yoga practitioners said they did yoga to promote health and support wellness; 48 percent said they did yoga to manage specific health conditions.

Because they are inherently gentle, mindfulness practices are low-risk exercise programs to begin as an older adult. There is also some benefit to coming to mindfulness practices when you are older, if you bring an intention of truly wanting to focus, a desire to be more introspective. Mindful fitness programs offer a low-threat way to promote health. As a culture, we may be uncomfortable talking about our stress, telling people our anxieties, but we can come to a yoga class without stigma, and learn breathing and focusing that then help us deal with our stress and anxiety. Mindfulness practices also support our sense of being self-sufficient and independent. They allow us to feel in control of our own care, our own well-being. And as we get older, that sense of feeling in control becomes more and more important.

Some people may be hesitant about trying mindful fitness programs; they may have their own religious or philosophical beliefs and be worried, if I try yoga, will it conflict with my religion. Mindfulness practices can actually enhance your own religious and philosophical beliefs. Several years ago, I taught a yoga class on Wednesday nights at a church, right before their Wednesday night service. We would end every class in silence, which allowed the participants to go straight into the service without distraction. Over a few weeks the class got larger and larger until I had 60 or 70 people in class every single week, and they shared that they kept coming and they brought their friends because the yoga class helped them to quiet their mind and focus their attention, so they felt that they were more present when they went into the worship service. They used the mindfulness practices to be more mindful, more fully in the moment, during their religious worship.

I will say not all mindfulness classes are suited to everyone, and a lot of it depends on the instructor. Some yoga teachers use Sanskrit or chanting; they have music, and incense in their classes, to give students a taste of the cultures out of which the practice arose. I don't use those in my classes as a deliberate decision because I want my students to focus on their breath, their movement, and their own experience, and not get stuck in a word or a technique that may make them uncomfortable or distracted. Also for many adults, background can interfere with hearing, and incense or scents may affect allergies or breathing issues like COPD. The point is that different instructors have different philosophical approaches to how they frame their class and how they teach mindfulness practices. If you find you want to learn more, you should know about this variety in teaching style. Try out different instructors; find the approach and the person who makes you most comfortable.

In this lecture, we will discuss several mindfulness practices: yoga, Tai Chi, and the martial arts. I also encourage you to try the chair yoga active session and the Qigong active session, so that you can experience the benefits of mindful fitness first hand.

The Sanskrit word *yoga* means "union." When we talk about yoga, what we are really talking about is an exercise practice that is intended to unify your mental and physical being. Yoga brings together physical and psychological exercise to cultivate both physical and psychological health and wellness. It is an exercise practice that is built on a cohesive philosophy, and which is now supported by solid empirical research. You could do psychological skills training and physical exercise as separate, isolated components. But with yoga, you have the opportunity to train both aspects of yourself in an integrated way.

While yoga has its background and history in the Indian tradition and the Hindu religion, yoga itself is a very pragmatic practice; it adapts to you, whatever your cultural, religious, or philosophical perspective. At its core, yoga is a practice intended to bring about unity of your mind and body. Through physical exercise, focused attention, and deliberate breathing, you can further a sense of connection between your internal and external self. Yoga is also uniquely effective in helping you manage and cope with stress.

How does it do that? There are two ways that yoga impacts your response to stress. First, a consistent yoga practice will, over time, reduce your reactivity to stress, both physiologically and psychologically. The common ways we physically manifest stress—rapid breathing, elevated heart rate, and muscular tension—are all improved through regular yoga practice. My own research has shown that just six weeks of yoga training helps increase self-control, and that this increased self-control may be related to improvements in other aspects of psychological well-being, such as anxiety and mood. Practicing yoga regularly makes stressful situations less likely to actually cause you stress.

Second, yoga provides a set of tools that you can use in response to stressful situations. When you practice yoga, you learn self-soothing skills that you can pull out as needed in a stressful situation. When stressors arise, you are more adept at handling them appropriately. You can step back, do a few minutes of yoga, and then approach the situation with a new, calmer perspective. In fact, even in a major crisis, yoga can be useful for helping you get through it. Researchers have found that just one week of yoga practice actually helped flood and tsunami victims recover more quickly and experience less stress by one month after the trauma.

The two ways yoga affects you can lead to powerful outcomes. The practice of yoga can physically change you. Magnetic Resonance Imaging studies show that it can actually change the structure of the brain, in particular, the amygdala, a part of the brain associated with stress. Yoga practice can change your hormone profile, and how your body processes the physiological effects of stress. Yoga can also improve lung function, even among those with asthma. Because yoga can help reduce inflammation in the body and help the body to be less reactive, regular yoga practice can even reduce symptoms of allergies.

In terms of preventative health, yoga can positively affect your blood glucose levels, your cholesterol levels, and your overall cardiovascular risk profile; this is true both in individuals with cardiovascular disease risk and in individuals with diabetes. Yoga is also beneficial for managing the stress that is often experienced as part of chronic and terminal illness. Among cancer patients, individuals with gastrointestinal diseases such as Irritable Bowel Syndrome and chronic pancreatitis, and individuals with chronic pain, research studies continually demonstrate yoga's potential for helping reduce the experience of stress and improve overall quality of life.

Let's say you've just gotten bad news, and you're feeling stressed and overwhelmed. In yoga theory, forward bends are considered protective, soothing, comforting; they take you within; they allow you to protect yourself, like a turtle going into his shell. Let's try one. Come and shit comfortably on a chair. Spread your legs wide, with your feet planted firmly into the floor. Hands start on your knees, chest is lifted, posture's open. Take a nice deep inhalation through your nose. Now exhale completely, letting all the stress and frustration come out of your body, and fold your body forward, down through your legs. Sink into that forward bend, stay down there, let your body relax into it. Feel yourself sinking deeper. Feel your breath coming gently in and out. Feel yourself becoming protected, safe, closing your shell in so that you have that moment to regain your sense of centeredness, your sense of being mindful in your body. Taking a few breaths there, just relax, inhaling and exhaling through the nose, letting your body sink forward and relax into your forward bend.

Now, we're gonna place the hands on the knees, gently push yourself to come back up to sitting. Relax your legs and take a few more deep breaths. Notice if you feel a little calmer, a little more contained, a little more grounded and centered. A forward bend is something simple that you can do anywhere, even at your desk at work, if you need to take your energy within and find a sense of internal quiet in the midst of a stressful day.

I have taught chair-based yoga in a variety of locations, because it's so adaptable. I have taught it in workplaces right after the workday, and the participants mostly came over in their work clothes and just removed their shoes. When I was in graduate school at Florida State University, I taught a free class at the Tallahassee Senior Center, and we did yoga in the cafeteria, right around the tables, right before lunch. My regulars always joined me for class, and each week I had a few new students who arrived early for lunch and decided, Why not? I'll give yoga a try.

So it's versatile, it's adaptable, and most importantly, it gives you new skills in your stress-management toolbox. First, you can practice yoga regularly to reduce your stress reactivity. Second, you can use the skills and exercises you learn as a quick reset whenever you're faced with an anxiety-provoking situation. For instance, people often tell you that when you're stressed you should take a few deep breaths. The problem is that when you're stressed, the breaths you take tend to be shallow and centered in your chest. Even if you think you're taking deep breaths, you're probably taking shallow, chest-based breaths that actually make your stress worse. If, however, you have been learning how to take deep, abdominal breaths as part of your yoga practice, you can actually take the kind of deep breaths that will help you work through a feeling of anxiety.

Let's contrast the way the two feel for a moment. First take two or three faux-deep breaths into your chest. Breathe in, and bring it into your chest the way you learned when you were young to take a deep breath. You're constricting your lungs in; you're not taking good, deep breaths. In contrast, place your hands on your belly and take three real deep breaths, down into the lower lobes of your abdomen, allowing your stomach to soften and relax. Inhale … exhale. Inhale … exhale. Again, one more. Inhale … exhale. Do you feel the difference in your body, in your breathing, and in your own sense of awareness between that shallow breathing and that slow, deep rhythmic breathing? At first, when you're learning new skills, it is challenging to put them into practice when you need them. Through ongoing practice of mindfulness skills, they feel more comfortable, and then you're able to use them when you need them.

Tai Chi and Qigong are another type of mindfulness practice; these are traditional forms of mindful exercise from China. *Qi* is the Chinese word for "energy" or "life force," and Chinese traditional medicine believes that energy flows through energy pathways in the body, called meridians. If your qi is blocked or unbalanced, this stagnant energy can lead to illness or injury. The practices of Tai Chi and Qigong are intended to support healthy energy flow, and thus to promote overall health and well-being. You may be familiar with acupuncture, which also works by promoting healthy energy flow through the meridians.

Also foundational to the philosophy of Tai Chi and Qigong is the idea of yin and yang, or opposites. The philosophical belief is that nature consists of opposing forces, yin and yang, in appropriate balance. Tai Chi and Qigong provide balanced yet opposite movements, open and closed, hard and soft, to support the appropriate equilibrium of yin and yang in your body. Tai Chi and Qigong are distinct practices, but they're often practiced together.

Tai Chi uses a specific series of movements, done as a meditation, to move qi in the body. You may have seen a Tai Chi class in the park. Many individuals like to practice outside, and the deliberate series looks like beautiful choreography. Qigong includes many different exercises, which may be done in different orders. It's often considered a foundational exercise to learn before you begin practicing the Tai Chi sequence. Movement is never forced, the muscles stay relaxed. The joints are never fully extended nor fully bent, so that the connective tissues are not stretched. The exercises can be adapted to whatever your fitness level.

The moves of Tai Chi and Qigong are so different from other forms of exercise because your movement is usually circular. So, for instance, instead of just stretching your arms straight out in front of you, you would keep your elbows and wrists soft as if you were hugging a gentle ball in front of you. If you were then moving your arm to the side you wouldn't just stick your arm out to the side, but rather you'd flow your arm out to the side. It's almost as if you are moving in water, where there is just a little bit of resistance, so it slows and softens the lines of your movement.

In 2009, the Harvard Women's Health Watch said that "while Tai Chi is often described as Meditation in Motion, it might well be called Medication in Motion" precisely because it is both so gentle and so beneficial for health. When we say that Tai Chi is meditation in motion, what we mean is that it is a form of meditative practice, of focusing your mind and your awareness through movement. Yoga is also a form of moving meditation. If you have a hard time sitting still, you may find that active forms of meditation like yoga and Tai Chi are more effective for you than seated meditation.

Tai Chi and Qigong promote health and well-being in many ways. First, they are great for helping you maintain or improve your posture, and supporting your balance. As we've discussed, balance is a key component of fitness as we age, to prevent falls. Tai Chi and Qigong are wonderful exercise forms as we age, because while they offer substantial health benefits, they're gentle on the joints, they're good for helping manage chronic pain. They support you moving gently and smoothly through full range of motion to help you maintain flexibility and your abilities for normal activities of living.

They also improve strength: Just 12 weeks may lead to a 30 percent increase in lower-body strength and a 25 percent increase in arm strength, almost as much of a strength increase as those who engage in resistance training. They also increase flexibility, improve balance, and reduce falls. Some interesting research has found that having a fear of falling can actually make you more likely to fall, and some studies have found that Tai Chi training in particular helps reduce the fear of falling.

There are a host of other benefits. For instance, because it is weight bearing, Tai Chi may help promote bone density. Because they help you manage and reduce stress, Tai Chi and Qigong can reduce risk for heart disease, lower blood pressure, and promote both quality and duration of sleep, even for individuals with insomnia. Because of how they support strength in your core-body muscles, Tai Chi and Qigong may be particularly helpful for improving balance and recovery after a stroke, even more so than other exercise programs. Likewise, for individuals with Parkinson's disease, even moderately severe Parkinson's disease, Tai Chi may help improve balance, walking ability, and overall well-being.

Tai Chi and Qigong have also been found to offer the kind of gentle movement that can help individuals with arthritis and fibromyalgia still exercise, and the practice may actually reduce perceptions of pain. Likewise, research has found that Tai Chi and Qigong practice can help promote better quality of life and the ability to carry out normal daily activities for individuals with cancer. Tai Chi and Qigong have also been found to boost immunity. For instance, shingles is a painful skin rash that older adults can contract due to a weakened immune system. One study indicated that the practice of Tai Chi and Qigong actually increase resistance to the shingles virus in older adults. Overall, like yoga, Tai Chi and Qigong can promote health and wellness through gentle movements, combined with deliberate focus and breathing exercises.

It can also be a social experience, and when people practice Tai Chi together it can look like a gentle, lovely, choreographed dance. A great way to experience Tai Chi is in a natural setting, and many cities offer Tai Chi sessions in parks during the warm weather months. You can try out a gentle Qigong-based workout in the active sessions, to get a sense for this practice, but I encourage you to seek out an instructor in your area to really get a full experience of what Qigong and Tai Chi can do for your mental and physical health. A systematic review of the research from the Department of Sports Medicine at Chengdu Sport University in China concluded that experience-based evidence indicates that martial arts may promote health and wellness, and that more research studies are warranted to validate those effects.

So I encourage you to surprise yourself, even if you've never thought about the martial arts. I took karate in college, and it was empowering. Early adulthood can be a tough, scary time, but somehow taking karate made me feel stronger, more in control, more ready to face the challenges that were ahead of me. At the same time my parents were going through an unpleasant divorce, and my mom was going through the self-esteem-battering experience of retirement plus menopause plus a divorce. On my summer break, I took her with me to karate classes, and she learned how to kick, and punch, and even broke boards with her hand and her foot. And it was really great for her. It gave her some of her fight back, some of her sense of belief in herself.

I want you to try for yourself how it can make you feel empowered, so let's do a quick demo. Stand up out of your chair. Take a nice wide stance, put your feet wide apart, firmly planted. Your knees are going to gently bend into a squat. Feel that your legs are strong and solid, connecting you to the earth. You're going to make fists, curling your fingers in, and then closing your thumbs on top. You never put your thumbs inside, because then if you actually punch something, you could break your thumb. Shoulders rolled down and back, elbows are bent, arms are gently at your side. Now we're going to take a nice deep inhalation, and then we're going to punch the right arm straight out, straight and strong, with a sharp, loud exhalation through the mouth. So you're going to breathe in, and—huwah—exhale out strong.

That strong exhalation is called the *kiai*, and it literally means "shout" or "spirit" in Japanese; it adds some force and power to your movement. Depending on the martial art, and the sensei, or instructor, you may hear it pronounced kiai, or hi-yah, or hu-uh, or even just a forceful grunt like hunn but the bottom line is that it is a forceful exhale through the diaphragm to increase the energy of your movement. We're going to take five punches, each side. Punch strong and follow through, keeping your squat steady and your posture solid. Each time you punch, return your opposite arm in toward your side, almost as if you are protecting your side. We're going to inhale, [punch], inhale [punch], and take whatever breath feels natural to you. Inhale [punch], inhale [punch]. Inhale [punch], inhale [punch]. Do one more. Inhale [punch]. And then just exhale your arms down to your sides, step your feet back together.

How do you feel? Do you have a sense of your own strength and power? Your energy? If you're going through a tough time, or if you've always been worried about being delicate and polite and careful, or maybe you're always feeling a little shy and quiet, maybe you're a little bit introverted, the martial arts are a great way to find that inner strength but in a controlled, centered, solid way, so you don't have to be overly energetic. You're just finding that energy that's already in you. Above all, the martial arts emphasize internal control, focus, and deliberate awareness. It is truly an active, moving meditation.

That being said, if you're going to try martial arts as a way to expand your horizons, talk to your doctor, and find the right instructor. Some instructors require sparring, which means you're actually practicing with other people. Others allow you to learn the *katas*, which are patterns or forms of movement, without having to make contact with others. Look for an instructor who will be mindful of your age and whatever health conditions you have, and then go forth and break the board, break your preconceived notions of what you can and can't do!

Meditation is always a part of mindfulness fitness practices, and if you attend a yoga, Tai Chi, or martial arts class you will spend some time practicing meditation. You can also practice meditation on its own. In a nutshell, meditation is focused awareness—deliberate training of the mind to reduce the ongoing jumble of thoughts that we live with most of the time. The renowned meditation teacher Jack Kornfield says that the mind is like a puppy; you are trying to train the puppy, and you put paper down, and the puppy wanders off and pees in the corner. You continue to pick the puppy up gently, and bring it back to the paper. And that's what our mind is like: We focus our awareness, and it wanders off somewhere else. Gently, we bring it back again. It wanders off again. We bring it back again. Through that process, that gentle but consistent retuning to deliberate focus, we learn to control our mind and our thoughts. And the process of learning control of your mind has powerful impacts.

Psychologically, meditation helps you gain perspective, manage stress, increase your sense of self-awareness, learn to focus on the present, and reduce negative emotions. It can also have profound impacts on our health. Research suggests that meditation can help with illnesses including allergies, asthma, heart disease and high blood pressure, even cancer. Meditation can also help with conditions that involve a sense of self-control, such as binge eating or substance abuse. I encourage you to try the two breath-based meditation practices offered in the active series of this course. They will give you a practical experience of the benefits of meditation. If you'd like to study meditation in more depth, The Great Courses also offers a full course on meditation, which includes both philosophical instruction and active practice sessions.

In this lecture, we've talked about mindfulness fitness practices: fitness programs that combine physical exercise with deliberate breathing and focused attention. Mindfulness practices include yoga, tai chi, and the martial arts, and they offer physical and psychological benefits beyond the benefits of just exercising. As we age, we begin to feel a divergence between a mind that remains young and a body that is beginning to show some of the effects of age. Mindfulness practices offer a gentle way to stay active, and psychologically they can help us to stay connected to our bodies, to help us compassionately accept the changes we experience with age.

Mindfulness doesn't come easily or naturally. It is a skill and a type of fitness; like any other component of fitness, it requires deliberate training and practice in order to cultivate it. I encourage you to try the active sessions on chair yoga, Qigong, and meditation, so that you can experience firsthand the techniques and the benefits of mindfulness practice.

For your takeaway activity, I'd like you to reflect on your current level of mindfulness. We'll do two activities in support of this. First, take 15 minutes for reflection on your thoughts, your inner awareness. Sit down by yourself in a quiet space with your journal and a pen. Set a timer for 15 minutes. Don't try to think of anything; don't try to focus on a particular topic, just let your mind wander. Jot down a few key words for each thought. Don't judge; don't try to direct, just become aware. Record your thoughts as they come without judging them. Jot down a few words to capture the stream of consciousness.

When you're done, look at what you've got. Your thoughts likely jumped around quickly from thing to thing: a task to complete at work, a fight with your spouse, something you need to buy at the grocery store, the windows that need to be cleaned, where you want to go on your vacation this year. Don't worry what they were, or what someone else would think; you're just doing this as an exercise in inner awareness, to learn how to become aware of your mind. We often don't even realize how our minds flutter, what movements go on, and this is a great exercise to gain that insight into your thoughts.

Next, pick a day and set a timer to go off every hour for that one day. Use your phone or your computer or an alarm on your watch. In your journal, make a chart with three columns labeled "past," "present," "future" and down the side, label each line for one hour of the day. Whenever your alarm goes off, write down one sentence to indicate what you're thinking about in the appropriate column. Are you thinking about the past, the present, or the future? Again, no judgments, no direction, just be aware and jot it down. At the end of the day look at the overall picture and assess how much time you spent in the past, how much time you spent in the future, and probably how little time you actually spent right here, in the here and now.

That's what mindfulness practices will help you learn: skills and strategies so that you can direct your mind to actually be right here, right now. In our next lecture, we'll continue our internal focus. We will talk more about how we can use self-awareness and self-understanding, specifically through goal setting and a better understanding of the limits of willpower, to support our successful outcomes.

Motivation—Goals and Willpower
Lecture 7

In Lecture 2, we focused on motivation, discussing the transtheoretical model and stages-of-change theory. In this lecture, we return to the topic of motivation again because it is vital to changing the way you live. You can't reap the benefits of exercise unless you actually do it. Probably the most important part of a successful exercise plan is figuring out your motivations and the strategies that will keep you motivated in the long run. In this lecture, we'll talk about SMART goals, that is, goals that are specific, measurable, attainable, realistic, and time-specific.

SMART Goals

- A goal is the ultimate aim toward which you direct effort. Well-thought-out goals motivate behavioral change; they define the destination and provide a road map for how to get there. SMART goals are those that are specific, measurable, attainable, realistic, and time-specific.

- To be achievable, a goal must be specific; it must include a definition of success. You can't just say, "I want to lose weight," because you won't know whether or not you've succeeded. A better, more specific goal is "I want to lose 10 pounds."

- In addition to being specific, a goal must also be measurable. You need to quantify the overall goal and the subcomponents you need to achieve to meet the goal.

- Goals must also be attainable for you. It's better to start small and move forward to greater goals with a feeling of success than to get discouraged because you failed to accomplish an unrealistic goal. Instead of setting a goal to run a marathon, decide that you will walk for 30 minutes 5 days a week. Once that becomes a habit, start jogging 3 days a week. By working through the smaller goals, you may eventually be able to achieve greater aspirations.

- A related quality of SMART goals is realism. Don't set yourself up for failure. For example, if you're short and naturally curvy, you may never have the figure of a supermodel, but you can still work out regularly to be fit and healthy. Realistic goals may focus more on the process ("I'll do resistance training for 20 minutes 3 days a week") than outcome ("I will fit into a size 4"). In setting realistic goals, also think about contingency plans. Can you do an alternative exercise if the weather prohibits you from walking outside?

- Finally, a SMART goal is time-specific. If you are setting an outcome-based goal, such as losing 10 pounds, establish a realistic time frame, such as 6 weeks, losing 1 to 2 pounds per week. If you are setting a process goal, choose a specific amount of time for which you will commit to the process, optimally, at least 6 weeks. Then, evaluate your progress and determine whether you should continue with the same goal or increase the requirements of the goal.

- In addition to the SMART components, you should also make sure to frame your goal positively. "I will eat oatmeal and berries for breakfast" is a good goal. "I will not eat donuts for breakfast" will just make you think about eating donuts. You should also write your goals down and look at them regularly and share your goals with a supportive friend or family member.

Willpower

- Though we like to think of ourselves as independent, autonomous people, the reality is that our environment affects us more than we know. And if your environment doesn't set you up for success, then you're relying on willpower—a limited resource—to push through in spite of the obstacles.

- One study at Florida State University showed that students who were forced to exercise their willpower to avoid temptation gave up on tasks much sooner than other students who had not been tempted. We seem to have limited quantities of willpower to work with, and every time we use our self-control, we draw from that

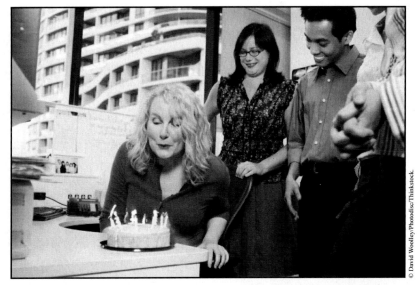

If you use your willpower to resist eating cake at an office birthday party, you may find that you've lost the willpower to work out at the gym on the way home.

resource. Further, when willpower is reduced through a distraction task, people are more likely to do things they would otherwise resist doing and to make irrational decisions.

- According to Stanford psychologist Kelly McGonigal, the biology of stress and the biology of willpower are incompatible. In other words, the more you suffer from chronic stress, the less willpower you have.

- Willpower is like a muscle, and you can support its development through practice, stress management, and sufficient sleep. Research has shown that when college students are given tasks that require self-control, such as tracking what they eat or using their weaker hands for the computer mouse, after a few weeks, they had greater willpower overall. Mindfulness practices can help in developing willpower because they are specifically focused on training the mind toward self-control.

Supportive Environments

- Set up your environment so that you aren't as reliant on willpower to make good decisions about diet and exercise. If you set up your environment in a supportive way, then you will have your willpower muscle ready and available in the situations where you really need its strength.

- For instance, if you live near a park or other open, natural space, you will be more physically active. If you have a window in your office that allows you to see green, natural space, you are less likely to experience work stress. If there is a supermarket in your neighborhood, you are more likely to eat at least five servings of fruits and vegetables each day. These environmental factors and others can have a significant impact on health-promoting decisions.

- Modern conveniences have eliminated a number of small opportunities to incorporate movement in everyday activities. Be aware of this fact and look for ways to bring that movement back into your environment.
  - Use a push lawnmower instead of a riding lawnmower or, even better, use a manual lawnmower and really get some exercise.

  - Ride a bike or walk when you run errands nearby, instead of driving your car.

  - Get in the habit of taking the stairs instead of the elevator or escalator.

  - Grate carrots or mix cookie batter by hand instead of using the food processor or mixer.

- Our social environments also influence our fitness and health-promoting decisions. For example, restaurants are colorful, well lit, and decorated in such a way as to encourage us to linger and eat more. Even experts can be taken in by the atmosphere in a restaurant; in one study, when trained dieticians were asked to estimate the nutrition information for five common restaurant meals, they underestimated calories by 37% and fat by 49%.

- You may not be able to move to a neighborhood with a local grocery store, tree-lined streets with sidewalks, and a park on every block, but you can still make small, tangible differences in your daily life through the way you structure your personal space.

  o For instance, you need to get sufficient sleep to manage stress, feel rested, and make good choices. If you have a TV or computer in your bedroom, move it to another room. Research shows that having an electronic device in your bedroom reduces both the quantity and quality of your sleep. If you're tired, you will have fewer reserves in your willpower muscle and you may make poor decisions.

  o Currently, Americans eat about 32% of our calories outside the home, but research shows that if you eat more meals at home, you are more likely to eat healthfully. At home, use your large dinner plates for salad and your salad plates for pasta or rice. This strategy gives you more appropriate portion sizes when you fill your plate.

  o You can also eat healthier by using fresh, whole foods and fewer packaged, processed foods. This approach instantly reduces the amount of hidden fat, sugar, and sodium you're consuming. You may think that you don't have time to cook fresh, whole food, but research from UCLA reports that cooking from scratch actually adds only about 10 extra minutes to meal preparation!

  o In your office, try bringing in a few potted plants and a natural-spectrum light if you don't have a window. You might also bring in some hand weights and stretch bands and do 5 or 10 minutes of strength training or stretching every hour or two. Pack your lunch instead of going out for fast food, and if the weather permits, take a short walk and eat outside.

- ○ Put your walking shoes and your dog's leash by the front door to encourage you to go for a walk instead of just putting the dog in the backyard.

- ○ Chop up fresh vegetables and prepare containers of salad on the weekends so you have some readily available snacks to grab when you're hungry during the week.

- Reconfiguring your environment for a healthier lifestyle may mean making many small changes, but doing so makes it much easier for you to make good choices—without relying on your limited willpower.

Suggested Reading

Baumeister and Tierney, *Willpower*.

McGonigal, *The Willpower Instinct*.

Activities and Assignments

Think creatively about how you can improve your environment to promote fitness. Consider physical changes in your home, modifications to your work environment or schedule, your commute, and your leisure activities, as well as your clothes, the food you keep in your house, lighting, and so on. Look for small improvements you can make in all aspects of your life to promote fitness and good health decisions.

Review your perspective on healthy aging from Lecture 1. Identify at least two components that are priorities. How can you make small, tangible decisions now to support those two components of healthy aging?

Set two SMART goals that connect environmental changes to promote your view of healthy aging. Remember, your goals should be specific, measurable, attainable, realistic, and time-specific.

Motivation—Goals and Willpower
Lecture 7—Transcript

Do you make New Year's resolutions? When's the last time you set one and actually kept it past the end of January? We have good intentions with our New Year's resolutions. We genuinely want to do better, to have a fresh start for the new year, to accomplish what we set out to accomplish. But when we say "I want to lose weight" or "I want to improve my marriage" or "I want to make more money" we are setting ourselves up for failure.

In Lecture 2, we focused on motivation, discussing the transtheoretical model and stages of change theory. Now, we are back to motivation again because it is so vital and so foundational. For all the benefits of exercise, for the strategies that you can apply, and the types of exercise you can try, none of it will come to anything if you don't actually do it. I truly believe that the most important part of a successful exercise plan is figuring out your motivations, and the strategies that will keep you motivated in the long run. In fact, I believe that motivation is such an important part of your exercise plan that we will come back to motivation yet again in our final lecture.

So, for motivation part 2, let's start by talking about goals. A goal is the ultimate aim towards which you direct effort. Goals motivate our behavioral change. When done well, goals define the destination and provide a road map for how to get there. To be effective, goals should be SMART, an acronym that stands for Specific, Measureable, Attainable, Realistic, and Time-specific. Let's look at each of the characteristics of a good goal in detail.

A goal should be specific. That means that to achieve a goal, you need to define what success looks like. For instance, let's look at the one that's on so many people's New Year's resolutions: I want to lose weight. How do you know if you've succeeded? If you lose one pound you've lost weight, but does that mean you've accomplished your goal? Does it mean a specific size? Does it mean you can fit back into the dress or suit you wore on your wedding day? Is it a favorite pair of jeans comfortably fastened around your waist? What do you actually mean when you say you want to lose weight? So, I want to lose weight is not a good goal because it's not specific. I want to lose 10 pounds is specific.

A goal should be measurable. This connects directly to specific: What does success look like, and how can you actually quantify it? Think about the specific subcomponents that you need to achieve the goal. These are your objectives. If it sounds a lot like annual performance evaluation, you're right; your human resource director is on the right track in asking you to set specific goals each year, including supportive objectives. Apply those same work principles to your own health and life, with measurable objectives.

A goal should be attainable. You are setting goals for you. Don't let someone else set them for you. This is not the time for pie-in-the-sky dreaming because when you fail to accomplish a goal, it can be discouraging, and that gets you off track for other health-promoting behaviors and other goals. Think about what you can really do. It's better to start small and move forward to bigger goals with a feeling of success, than to have to backtrack because you didn't achieve your goal.

Maybe you want to run a marathon, but if you're not working out at all, a marathon is a lofty goal. Put it on your bucket list, but focus your goal right now on walking for 30 minutes five days a week. Once that's easy, set the goal for jogging three days a week, and then ramp up to running, and then start increasing your time. Take it one step at a time, and start with the hill right in front of you. The mountain in the distance is aspiration, but for principles of goal setting, be specific and focus on the attainable task in front of you. Success leads to success, and when you get to the foot of the mountain, you'll have success, and self-confidence, and good solid skills to help you conquer that goal when it's time.

You also need to think about what is really attainable for your life, right now. Maybe you'd love to try club sports. Your local adult soccer league practices four days a week from 4–6 pm. If you have kids in school and activities, that probably interferes with school pick-up, so joining the soccer league right now is probably not attainable. Playing on a community soccer team can stay on your list of aspirations, but it's not a good goal for right now, because it doesn't fit into the parameters you are currently working with. Perhaps right now your focus is on working up to running comfortably for an hour, four days a week, and then when your schedule opens up, you'll be able to keep up on the soccer field.

A goal should be realistic. Realistic connects to attainable, and maybe when we talk about goals we emphasize this twice precisely because it is so important, and because people so often set themselves up for failure with unrealistic goals. Say you're like me, a woman who is 5'4", naturally curvy, childbearing hips, my grandma would have said. You can set a goal to work out regularly, to be fit and strong and healthy. But lean and leggy, I am never going to be.

So when you're thinking realistically about your goals, focus in on those things that are specific and measurable because that's where you'll find realistic success. What you'll find is that if you are working on a goal that is specific, realistic, and measurable, most of the time, you'll be talking about process goals, not outcome goals. So this is where we will take a different approach from what your human resources department asks you to do during your annual work objective planning process.

What I mean is that while "I will lose five pounds" is measurable, specific, realistic, it's focused on an outcome. A better approach is to set goals about your process, goals like: I will do resistance training for 20 minutes, three days a week. I will take a refillable bottle of water to work, and sip it throughout the day, so that I've drunk 64 ounces of water before I go home. I will turn my television and electronics off one hour before bedtime, so that I have some relaxing downtime before bed. I will eat a fresh salad with at least two fresh vegetables as my first course for dinner at least five nights a week. Those goals are about the process, about what you're doing. In this course, we are focusing on the process of doing healthy things so that you feel better and feel more fit and feel more healthy.

I can't guarantee that you'll feel better about yourself, or feel happier and healthier, if you are five pounds lighter. There is actually some evidence that you might not. There are some published memoirs of individuals who lost substantial amounts of weight, only to discover that their problems and their dissatisfaction were still waiting for them in the closet, right next to their skinny jeans. But making positive, health-promoting, small decisions every day, those will have an impact on how you feel. Like dominoes, they'll help promote other health-promoting decisions, which will also have an impact on how you feel.

When you're thinking about realistic goals, also think about contingency plans. For instance, if you set a goal that you will walk for 30 minutes, five days per week, and you live in North Dakota and January comes along, what are you going to do when a blizzard hits? What is an acceptable solution that will help you stay on track and feel like you're meeting your goals? Maybe an exercise DVD you can do? Maybe you can shovel snow? Walk in place while you watch television? Bundle up and head out with either snowshoes or cross-country skis? Build those contingency plans into your objectives and your goal, so that you have as many opportunities for success as possible.

A goal should also be time specific. If you are setting an outcome-based goal (the "I will lose five pounds" goal) set a timeframe that is realistic. Losing 1–2 pounds per week is realistic for long-term weight loss. If you are setting the process goals, set a specific amount of time for which you will commit to the process. According to research published in the *European Journal of Social Psychology*, for 95 percent of individuals, it takes between 18 and 254 days to fully adopt a new behavior and make it automatic. So it will take you between one and eight-and-a-half months to turn a good behavior into a habit. That's a lot of variation, based on individual personality. You should assess yourself, look at your past successes, figure out the right amount of time for you. But set a goal to do your new behavior consistency for at least six weeks, and then you can evaluate and determine whether you should continue with the goal, change the goal, or increase the requirements of the goal.

A few other aspects of goal setting that you may find helpful, include that you should frame your goal positively. For instance, "I will eat oatmeal and berries for breakfast" is a good goal. "I will not eat donuts for breakfast" is not a good goal because it's just going to make you think about the donuts. You should also write your goals down and look at them regularly. The mind has a way of playing tricks on you—did I say five days a week or did I say four?—and that can sabotage your progress. You should also share your goals with someone whom you trust to be supportive, but avoid talking about your goals with someone who may unconsciously or consciously interfere. We'll talk more about social support and how friends can both help and hurt our healthy lifestyles in our next lecture.

It's important to think clearly about what we want to accomplish, so that we can set up our environment in a way that supports our success. Though we like to think of ourselves as independent, autonomous people, the reality is that our environment affects us more than we know. Your environment has a strong impact on the decisions you make. If your environment doesn't set you up for success, then you're relying on willpower to push through in spite of the obstacles. While we often look at people who are fit and healthy and assume that they have strong willpower, research shows that willpower is actually a limited resource. You can't count on your willpower to push you through to a healthy decision every time.

Let me give you a research example. Roy Baumeister, a research psychologist at Florida State University, focuses much of his work on understanding willpower. In one study, he asked college students to fast, to not eat anything. Then, they were invited into a laboratory waiting room with a table of chocolate, fresh chocolate chip cookies, and radishes. The cookies had been baked in the lab, so the lab smelled like the fresh chocolate chip cookies. Some students were invited to eat the cookies or the candy. Other students, poor dears, were told that they could only eat the radishes. The researchers left the room, and observed through a hidden window. The radish students struggled: They smelled the cookies, they gazed longingly at the cookies, some students even picked them up, but not one radish student actually ate a cookie. Students were escorted into another room, and given puzzles to solve—puzzles that couldn't actually be solved.

One group of students also came in fasting and was immediately taken to the puzzles, without any of the temptation of cookies or cookie smells. The students who had eaten candy or cookies, and the students who were not tempted by the presence of candy or cookies, worked for about 20 minutes trying to solve the puzzles before they gave up. The students who had to resist the cookies and resign themselves to radishes gave up in just eight minutes. They had used their willpower up on the cookies; they didn't have any left for the puzzles.

In another study, when participants were asked to stifle their emotional response when watching a sad video, they were less able to persist on a hand-gripping task. Another study at a car dealership found that buyers were more deliberate, more effortful, on their first few decisions. So practically, when you go to a car dealer, talk about important things first. If you use up all your emotional energy picking paint color and interior fabric, you may be less likely to make good decisions about potentially more costly choices later on in the process.

We have limited quantities of willpower to work with, and every time we use our self-control, we draw from the same energy source. Research has found that when willpower is reduced through a distraction test—avoiding the temptation of fresh cookies, trying not to cry at a sad movie, or trying not to laugh at a comedy clip—people are more likely to do lots of things that they would otherwise resist doing. People in committed relationships are more likely to look at attractive members of the opposite sex or to fight with their spouse, people are more likely to express prejudice, they are less likely to compromise, and they are more likely to make irrational decisions. One psychologist has actually proposed that this limitation of our willpower reserves may make marriage more challenging for dual-working couples. He poses that if you use all of your willpower and energy to behave well at work, you may be out of willpower by the end of the day, and find yourself angry and irritated at your spouse for every little thing.

When we talk about health-promoting decisions, this means that if we spend all of our willpower at work, we may be out of willpower by the time we leave the office. If you use your willpower to avoid the donuts in the office kitchen at breakfast, the cake at the office party at lunch, and the peanuts and greasy chips at the bar during the office happy hour, plus you withhold your opinion when you disagree with your boss or a colleague, you may well use up all the willpower you've got. Even though you mean to go to the gym on the way home, you'll skip it due to fatigue, and you'll find yourself eating junk food and watching TV on your couch, when you know you'd feel better eating a salad and going to bed a little earlier.

Stress in particular reduces our capacity for willpower. We talked in Lecture 3 about stress and how stress impacts the body. According to Stanford psychologist Kelly McGonigal, the biology of stress and the biology of willpower are incompatible. So the more you suffer from chronic stress, the less willpower you have. If you're sleep deprived, even if you're getting six hours a night, which so many busy people think of as normal, the effects on your brain are about the same as being a little bit drunk. And as you know, when you're a little bit drunk, you make poor decisions about food and social interactions and other things that require the kind of self-control that is implicit in will power.

Willpower is like a muscle, and you can support the development of willpower through practice, stress management, and sufficient sleep. You need to be well rested in order to make good decisions and have sufficient mental energy to make them. You can also build more of the willpower muscle by exercising your willpower. Baumeister's research at Florida State has shown that when college students are given tasks that require self-control—f or instance, tracking what they eat, or exercising regularly, or using their weaker hand for their computer mouse, or carefully watching their speech to only use full sentences and avoid profanity—after a few weeks, they had greater willpower overall: They smoked, drank, and snacked less, watched less television, studied more, and even washed their dishes more regularly! They were also more resistant to having their willpower depleted in laboratory experiments. Your willpower is a muscle, and you can build it by practicing, and by reducing your overall stress level through stress management, physical exercise, sufficient sleep, and good nutrition. Mindfulness practices can also help, since they specifically focus on training the mind toward self-control.

You can also set your environment up in a way to support good decisions. This way you aren't as reliant on willpower to make good decisions about diet, exercise, and health. If you set up your environment in a supportive way, then you will have your willpower muscle ready and available in the situations where you really need its strength. Let's talk, now, about how your environment impacts your health and your health-promoting decisions. For instance, if you live near a park or another open, natural space, you will be more physically active. If you have a window in your office that allows you to see green, natural space, you are less likely to experience work stress.

As you get older, if you live in an area with sidewalks and park access, you may actually live longer. If there is a supermarket in your neighborhood, you are more likely to eat at least five servings of fruits and vegetables each day. Even nuances like the patterns of the sidewalks in your neighborhood can have an impact. If your neighborhood has streets in a grid pattern, you are more likely to walk than if your neighborhood has lots of dead-ends and cul-de-sacs.

Culture can impact what our environment looks like. In the United Kingdom, street-design manuals indicate that there should be sidewalks on both sides of the street, but American street-design manuals recommend sidewalks on one side of the street only. These cultural differences can impact our preferred modes of transportation. In Austria, the Netherlands, Denmark, Italy, and Sweden, walking and biking account for between 40 and 54 percent of all daily trips. In the U.S., the automobile accounts for 84 percent of all daily trips, and walking and biking are only 10 percent of trips.

In Lecture 5, we discussed how we can leverage the activities of daily living into physical fitness. As we talk about environmental factors, let's consider for a moment how improvements in modern-day society have actually reduced our fitness, and how we can choose to be more active. You can probably guess the big ones: You could use a push lawnmower instead of a riding lawnmower, or even better, you could get an old-fashion manual lawnmower and really get some exercise. If you can make it work, you could ride a bike or walk for nearby errands, instead of driving your car.

But even those kinds of decisions can be challenging. For instance, you should take the stairs instead of the elevator or escalator. And you should, but it's not always easy in practice. The next time you go to a shopping mall, see if you can even find stairs in most two-floor department stores. There is probably one obvious set of stairs in the center of the mall but it's right by the food court, so then you've got the challenge that you've promoted exercise by using the stairs, but you're setting yourself up for unneeded snacking by throwing all those smells and scents and samples, all that temptation at yourself. And the last thing you want to do is reduce your willpower by searching for stairs just before you walk through a haven of fatty, greasy, junk food! There are also a lot of little conveniences every day, that don't seem like much, but 1- and 2- and 5- and 10-calorie decisions all day long can really add up.

For instance, do you remember when you actually had to crank down your car window? That burned a couple of calories every time you opened it, and every time you closed it. I have two kids and a minivan, so every time I get ready to load the kids in, I push a button on my key fob, and the side doors open up all by themselves. When I was a teenager, I actually had to muscle a heavy door open that didn't have any automation to it; that was a couple of calories anytime I drove my car. Have you ever mashed potatoes or grated carrots by hand instead of just popping them in the food processer? Five to 10 calories right there. Think about all the small conveniences you have now that used to be things that you actually had to move to accomplish.

Our social environments also influence our fitness and health-promoting decisions. The environment encourages it. The food industry spends $33 billion a year on advertising. Restaurants are colorful, well lit, and decorated on purpose in ways that encourage us to stay, buy more, and eat more. They give us free drink refills because that keeps us lingering and then we buy dessert. Even experts are taken in; in one study, trained dieticians were asked to estimate the nutrition information for five common restaurant meals. These trained dieticians underestimated calories by 37 percent and underestimated fat by 49 percent.

And most of us, 69 percent of Americans, according to one study by the American Institute for Cancer Research, will clean our plate and eat what we're served, regardless of portion size. And our portion sizes have gotten bigger, to keep up with our plates. In 1900, the average dinner plate had a 9-inch diameter. By 1950, the average dinner plate had a 10-inch diameter. By 2010, 12 inches was the standard diameter for the dinner plate in America. So we use bigger plates, we put more food on them, and we still clean our plates.

Interestingly, the extra food doesn't actually make us feel better. In one study, when people were given different sizes of sandwiches, the participants given larger sandwiches ate more. But there were no differences in how hungry or full they felt, regardless of the size of the sandwiches. And we eat more and then don't make up for the extra calories later. In another study, the size of a snack had no impact on how much food people ate at their next meal. But those bigger portions add up: 50 additional calories per day adds up to 5 additional pounds per year. Five extra pounds a year, from food that we don't even notice, and that doesn't actually make us feel more satisfied.

So what can you do? You may not be able to move to a neighborhood with a local grocery store, tree-lined streets with sidewalks, and a park on every block, but you can still make small, tangible differences in your daily life through the way you structure your personal space. You want to make it easy for you to choose fitness and health-promoting decisions. For instance, you need to get sufficient sleep to manage your stress, feel rested, and make good choices. So if you have a TV or computer in your bedroom, I've said it before, move it to another room. Research shows that having an electronic device in your bedroom reduces both the quantity and quality of your sleep. If you're tired, you make poor decisions. If you're tired, you have fewer reserves in your willpower muscle.

We talked in this lecture about food portions and plate size. Currently, as Americans we eat about 32 percent of our calories outside of our homes. Those are usually not nutrient-dense calories. Research shows that if you eat more of your meals at home, you are more likely to eat healthfully. When we're eating at home, because we dish our food based on the size of our plate, we can help ourselves out by using appropriately sized plates. So swap up your table setting use your large dinner plate for your salad and fill the plate up, and use your salad plate for your pasta or rice, so that when you fill your plate and clean it, it's a more appropriate portion size.

You can also eat healthier by using fresh, whole foods and less prepackaged, processed foods, because you'll instantly reduce the amount of hidden fat, sugar, and sodium you're consuming. You may think that you don't have time to use fresh, whole food but research from the UCLA Center on the Everyday Lives of Families reports that cooking from scratch actually only adds about 10 extra minutes to meal preparation! It may be that families who cook at home using more prepared, convenience foods end up overcompensating. They make more options at each meal, and essentially eliminate the time saved by so-called convenience foods.

Let me give you a personal example about how environment can affect you. Early in my academic career, I worked in a small cubicle in a basement office, with no windows and no natural light. So I had to make deliberate decisions to make my workspace healthier. I brought in potted plants, a small fan, and two natural spectrum lights to make my cubicle seem healthier and greener and more airy. I brought in some hand weights and some stretch bands that I kept under my desk, and I did 5–10 minutes of strength training or stretching every hour or two, just to get up from my desk and move around.

I brought my lunch, and focused on fresh vegetables and whole grains. I kept a case of water in my office. At lunchtime, I found a small park about 10 minutes away, and whenever I could I'd would walk out to the park and eat lunch on a park bench, and that 15 or 20 minutes of sunshine and fresh air and the walk, helped make a difference. I also lived only a few miles from my office on campus, so whenever the weather permitted, I walked to and from work, to get some more sunshine and fresh air.

It took a lot of small decisions to make me feel healthier when I was working in an environment that didn't feel healthy. But by setting up those decisions in consistent environmental ways, I made it easy on myself to make good choices. The good choices became easy because of how I restructured the environment. So that's what we have to do: think about how to make good choices easy with ways we can restructure our environment, given the environmental constraints that we have.

So take a look at your own life, your own constraints, and think about what choices can you make to set up your life to promote your health and wellness. How can you improve your environment so that you can maximize your willpower for when you really need it? Can you set your walking shoes and your dog's leash by the front door so it's easy to take him for a walk, instead of just putting him in the backyard? Can you pack your lunch for work every day so that instead of waiting in line at a fast food restaurant, you have a lunch that is faster and healthier? Maybe even pack your lunch while you're making dinner, to make it that much easier. Can you chop up fresh veggies on weekends and have containers of salad in your fridge, so that it's fast and simple to grab carrots and hummus when you get home from work hungry? Think about these kinds of small decisions, simple changes, so that your environment helps, instead of hurts, you and your health.

For this lecture's takeaway, first I'd like you to think deliberately and creatively about how you can improve your environment to support and promote fitness. What physical changes can you make in your house to make exercise an easy decision? What changes can you make in your schedule? How can you modify your workday, your commute, or your weekend activities? Think about changes that will support you by making exercise and health-promoting activities simple and easy so that you don't use up your valuable will power.

Next, go back to your first list, from Lecture 1, about what healthy aging means to you. Identify at least two components of that vision of healthy aging that are high priorities. How can you work on them now, in small, manageable, ways? For instance, do you want to feel more rested? Do you want to feel less stressed? Do you want to be more active?

I'd like you set two SMART goals that connect your vision of healthy aging to tangible changes you can make in your environment. For instance, if you want to feel more rested and less stressed, sleep is a great place to start. You move your television and computer out of your bedroom, and you set a goal to be in bed by 10 pm five nights a week. Define the goal according to your SMART principles: Specific, Measurable, Attainable, Realistic, and Time-specific. Set supportive objectives that will help you achieve the goal.

Commit to the goal for at least six weeks before you reevaluate – and remember, that it can take as much as eight-and-a-half months for that new habit to really set in. That's why I want you to connect your goal to something you can change in your environment to support you achieving the goal. By combining a clear, supportive goal-setting exercise with an environmental support system, you're providing yourself your best chance for success.

And that's what this whole course is about. The reality is that health and fitness are important, they are foundational, and they are deceptively simple. They seem easy. We all know they're important. But really, especially due to our limited capacity for will power, they're hard. We need as many tools, as many resources, and as many support systems as possible to help us succeed. You can do it.

Friends, Fitness, and Social Support
Lecture 8

Consider how many times in the past week you've combined social interactions with calorie consumption—happy hour with colleagues, dinner out with your spouse, or coffee and donuts with a friend. It seems natural and comfortable to share food and drinks with our family and friends, but we rarely share fitness activities with them. In childhood, fitness is often an opportunity for social interaction; children play outdoor games with their friends, ride bikes, or go swimming, but at some point, as adults, our social activities come to focus on eating and drinking. In this lecture, we'll see how social relationships can support, promote, and even inspire health and fitness and how fitness activities can support and cultivate friendships.

Benefits of Social Relationships

- Having strong social relationships is important for overall health. In fact, in terms of risk for premature death, having a low level of social interaction is more harmful than not exercising, twice as harmful as being obese, and as harmful as smoking 15 cigarettes a day or being an alcoholic. When we have connections with other people, we have a greater sense of purpose, and that can help us feel motivated to take better care of ourselves and to take fewer health risks.

- People who report that they are lonely report the same number of stressful life events as non-lonely people, but they report higher levels of chronic stress and indicate more feelings of helplessness and threat. Lonely people also experience loneliness physiologically; they have higher concentrations of stress hormones in their urine and sleep more poorly at night.

- If you feel lonely or isolated, you already know that situation has a negative impact on your life. If you're the primary caretaker for a loved one, you may feel so pressed for time that you don't have space or energy to cultivate relationships. But you don't have to become a social butterfly; what you need is just a few close friends you can count on.

Social Factors in Weight Gain and Loss

- Researchers have long noted that among children, obese students tend to be in the same social circles as other obese students.

  ○ A longitudinal study of high school students reported that some of this effect may be the result of a tendency to bond with people perceived as similar to oneself, but some of it is due to influence.

  ○ When students who were borderline overweight were friends with students who were active and lean, they were 40% more likely to decrease their BMI over the course of a school year. In contrast, if they were friends with students who were obese, they were 56% more likely to increase their BMI in the same year. The friends influenced such decisions as watching TV versus playing active sports.

- Research with adults also supports the evidence that weight gain is socially contagious. A large-scale analysis of more than 12,000 adults over 32 years tracked the relationship between obesity and social relationships. Interestingly, friends are more powerful in this regard than family. If your spouse becomes obese, your chance of obesity goes up by 37%. If your sibling becomes obese, your likelihood goes up by 40%. But if your friend becomes obese, your likelihood goes up by 57%.

- On the positive side, research has also shown that when one person loses weight, his or her friends and family are more likely to lose weight, too. In a statewide initiative in Rhode Island, a weight-loss campaign found that a team approach led to better outcomes. People who lost at least 5% of their initial body weight tended to be on the same team, and high levels of teammate social influence increased odds of clinically significant weight loss by 20%.

- One caveat with regard to social networks and weight-loss outcomes is this: If you are the first to lose weight or if your weight loss may change the social order, friends and family may unconsciously sabotage your weight-loss efforts. You may even unconsciously sabotage your own weight-loss efforts to return social relationships to "normal." In one large survey, 24,000 overweight women reported that losing weight created problems in their relationships that regaining the weight resolved.
  - If your friends and family are sabotaging your weight-loss efforts, they probably don't even realize they're doing it. And even if they want to help, they might not know how, or they might have their own beliefs that make it hard for them to understand what you're doing.

  - At the Duke University Diet and Fitness Center, after a 3-week in-patient program, participants write a "Dear Supporter" letter to take home to friends and family that communicates the help needed. You might think about using a similar approach to express to your friends and family how they can help with your weight-loss efforts.

- As we've said, it can be challenging to make a conscious decision in the right direction because there are unconscious clues in the environment that affect our eating decisions. We all usually think that we're independent individuals who are capable of making good decisions, but experimental studies show that we're not as good at understanding unconscious motivation as we think we are.
  - In one study, individuals walking through a lobby were randomly stopped and asked to complete a survey. The surveys had photographs of an overweight individual, a normal-weight individual, and a lamp.

  - After completing the survey, subjects were told they could help themselves to a bowl of candy. Those who were exposed to the picture of the overweight individual took an average of 30% more candy!

- Interestingly, research also shows that when we eat with others, we match our portion size to social norms. We may eat more or less than we normally would based on what others are eating. Researchers suggest that if you tend to eat small portions, you should eat meals by yourself, because the social norms in group eating may cause you to choose larger portions. If you tend to overeat, you should eat meals with others, because the social norms may help you to choose smaller portion amounts.

Social Factors in Fitness Behaviors

- Social norms are powerful forms of control over human behavior. If you're trying to incorporate health-promoting behaviors into your life, the key is to determine how to use your social environment to support those behaviors.

- For instance, 90% of exercise program participants prefer to exercise with a partner or group than to exercise alone. And self-determination theory holds that one of the primary motivators for human behavior is connectedness. If you establish a fitness program that helps you feel connected to others, you are more likely to stick with it.

- If your fitness program helps foster your sense of connection, then you're getting multiple benefits: You feel better, you get physical health benefits, and the program supports your relationships. In addition, the sense of commitment to another person may keep you going even when your motivation lags. This holds true in families, as well. Research studies have found that maternal and paternal exercise levels can predict a child's activity levels.

- Though marriage is often shown to increase health and promote longevity, the impact of marriage may depend on the health of your spouse. If your spouse has poor health, you are more likely to smoke cigarettes and less likely to exercise. In contrast, if you are married and join a fitness program by yourself, the likelihood that you will drop out is 43%, but if you join with your spouse, the likelihood you will drop out is only 6.3%!

Fostering Social Relationships

- Ironically, just as we're learning how important our social networks are for health, we find ourselves increasingly isolated. From 1985 to 2004, the mean number of people with whom Americans say they can discuss important matters dropped from 2.94 to 2.08. The number of people who say they have no one to discuss important matters with more than doubled in the same two decades, up to 25%.

- Researchers have different theories about why our social networks are becoming smaller and more fragile. In the modern world, people move more often, which breaks up the social networks into which we were born. Many of us also work more, which means that more of our waking hours are spent either at work or at home. Even when we're not technically working, many of us still monitor work on mobile devices.

- It's important to take a close look at opportunities for interaction in your own life. Is your schedule packed with paid work, caretaking of children or parents, and household chores? Are you on an electronic leash even when you're away from work? If you add in necessary daily tasks, such as sleeping, showering, and eating, you'll find you don't have much time left for social interactions.

Parents may find that their teenagers are inclined to open up more if they're involved in an activity rather than being forced to talk over the dinner table.

  o Further, you may be spending the little leisure time you have online. Survey results show that the average American spends 2 hours a day on social networking and that those who regularly use social networking sites spend 3.8 hours a day making virtual connections.

- Although those virtual connections can lead to broader social networks, deeper relationships still require face-to-face interaction.

- Many of us are saving money for our retirement years, but are we also taking time to build and nurture the relationships that we will need to have a happy retirement? If all of your friends are at work, what happens if you lose your job, become ill and have to take time off, or retire? Of course, positive relationships at work or online matter, but it's also important to build a social network in the real world and outside of work for true fitness and wellness.

- It's more difficult to make friends as we get older; people have obligations that make building relationships challenging. You have to be as deliberate about cultivating relationships as you are about cultivating other aspects of your health and wellness. Make an effort to find opportunities to connect with other people. Fill your life with activities you enjoy, causes you believe in, and places you like to be so that you'll have the chance to meet people who have similar interests.

- Relationships and social norms have a powerful impact on health and fitness, and there are many ways to put that power to good use. Take your parents out for a walk when you visit them; instead of dinner and a movie with your spouse, opt for a dance class; go outside with your children or play an active video game with them; meet your friends for a golf game; or take a family vacation at a national park. Think about how you can build relationships through fitness—and how you can get fit through relationships.

Suggested Reading

Carrol and Kimata, *Partner Yoga.*

Christakis and Fowler, *Connected.*

Kasl, *If the Buddha Dated.*

————, *If the Buddha Married*.

Paul, *The Friendship Crisis*.

Richo, *How to Be an Adult in Relationships*.

Activities and Assignments

Assess the support of your friends and family. Do you have friends and family who could be considered health-promoters? If so, how can you better connect with them and ask for their support? Do you have friends who may be unconsciously sabotaging your health and well-being? If so, what can you say to them to help them understand why you are making these changes, and how can you help reduce their sense of being threatened? How can you adapt the relationship to improve the friendship while you are improving your health?

Assess the degree to which your social network is connected to work. How can you consciously expand your social network beyond the workplace?

Think about other social opportunities you could seek out. In what ways can you connect the ones you love with the healthy lifestyle you are working to build?

Friends, Fitness, and Social Support
Lecture 8—Transcript

I'd like to start with a reflection, so grab your journal. Now take a minute and tally up how many times in the past week you've combined social interactions with calorie consumption. Catching up over a cup of coffee, happy hour with friends or colleagues, an intimate dinner with a loved one, an office party with cake or bagels. Now, take a minute and think about if you've had even one deliberate incidence of social interactions combined with calorie burning in the last week? Why is that? Why do we consider it so natural, so comfortable, so common to share food and drinks with our friends and family, and yet it's so rare to share our fitness with them?

And contrast that picture, that framework, to your childhood. When you were a kid did you ever walk across town to your best friend's house to ask him to go out to eat or go grab a cup of coffee? No! We went to our friends and asked if they could come out and play hide and seek or hopscotch or catch, ride bikes, go swimming, play stickball in the street. We got together for games of kickball and tag. In the summer, we got into swimsuits in the morning and stayed in the water playing Marco Polo until our parents made us come home for dinner. Maybe at the end of a long day, your friend's mom asked if you wanted to stay for dinner, but that was a side effect.

We used to look at fitness as fun, as something we did with our friends, something that we did to meet the opposite sex, even, with dates at the roller-skating rink or the bowling alley! It was something we found fun and engaging and exciting and relationship building. We woke up in the morning bounding with energy and ready to run and jump and play and explore with our friends. When did that stop? At what age did our friendships become about sitting around and eating, instead of exploring the world together? Why do we have this adult conception that good conversations happen while we're still and sitting and have a drink in our hands?

So that's what I'd like to talk about in this lecture: the intersection of our relationships and our fitness decisions. Because they are connected, and in fact, they are reciprocal. Your relationships can support, promote, even inspire your health and fitness, and your fitness activities, can support, improve, and even cultivate friendships and relationships. In fact, I would like you to expand your conception of fitness and consider that social relationships are a part of your fitness. Having strong social relationships is important for your health. In fact, in terms of risk for premature death, having a low level of social interaction is more harmful than not exercising, twice as harmful as being obese, and as harmful as smoking 15 cigarettes per day or being an alcoholic. When we have connections with other people, we have a greater sense of purpose, and that can help us feel motivated to take better care of ourselves, and to take fewer health risks.

People who report that they are lonely report the same number of stressful life events as non-lonely people, but they report higher levels of chronic stress and indicate more feelings of helplessness and threat. Lonely people also experience that loneliness physiologically; they have higher concentrations of stress hormones in their urine, and sleep more poorly at night. If you are feeling lonely or isolated, you already know that it is having a negative impact on your quality life. If you're in the middle of caretaking for a loved one, you may feel so pressed for time that you don't have space or energy to cultivate relationships right now. The intent of this lecture is not to make you feel bad about yourself for having a narrow social network, but rather to give you some new motivations to help you break out of your shell, and some suggestions and strategies for how to get started, when you're ready. We're not trying to turn an introvert into an extrovert; we're not trying to transform a shy flower into a social butterfly. You don't need to change your life and have a gaggle of friends, but it is important for you to have at least a few true blue souls whom you can really count on. Let's look at social relationships as one additional component of wellness, so that you have a holistic view of how to stay fit as you age.

Remember our centenarians? As we discussed earlier, the three specific health-promoting characteristics they share are they exercise regularly, they maintain a positive mental attitude, and they maintain a good social network. And those three components are interwoven. Because as we've discussed, regular exercise improves psychological health, so when you exercise regularly, you are more likely to have a positive mental attitude. It's also likely that success breeds success—so you exercise, and that helps you have a more positive attitude, and that positive attitude makes you more likely to see the benefits of exercise and to get up regularly to do it.

Your social network affects both your attitude and your exercise behaviors. In fact, weight gain may be socially contagious. Researchers have long noted that among kids, obese students tend to be in the same social circles as other obese students. A longitudinal study of high school students reports that some of this effect may be due to a tendency to bond with people like you. But some of it is due to influence. When students who were borderline overweight were friends with students who were active and lean, they were 40 percent more likely to decrease their body mass index over the course of one school year. In contrast, if they were friends with students who were obese, they were 56 percent more likely to increase their body mass index in that same year. The friends influenced decisions like screen time and playing active sports. So weight gain is contagious in that you "catch" the behaviors of your friends, and those behaviors affect your own decisions and behaviors, which impact your waistline.

Research with adults also supports the evidence that weight gain is socially contagious. A large-scale analysis of more than 12,000 adults over 32 years tracked the relationship between obesity and social relationships. Interestingly, friends are more powerful than family. If your spouse becomes obese, your chance of obesity goes up by 37 percent. If your sibling becomes obese, your likelihood goes up by 40 percent. If your friend becomes obese, your likelihood goes up by 57 percent.

Siblings and friends of the same sex had the greatest impact on your weight outcomes. So if you are a woman and your sister gains weight, that has more of an impact on you than if your brother does. The friends and family members had an influence even if they lived hundreds of miles away. Immediate neighbors who weren't close friends did not have an influence, so maybe it's not so much that we're keeping up with the Joneses, as we are keeping up with the people we love. And the big decisions we make with our friends and family, particularly, how we spend our leisure time, and whether we fill family time with food or activity, can have big impacts on our waistline.

Positively, the research showed that when one person lost weight, their friends and family were more likely to lose weight, too. Your social network can play a significant role in your weight loss. In a statewide initiative in Rhode Island, a weight-loss campaign found that a team approach to weight loss led to greater outcomes; people who lost at least five percent of their initial body weight tended to be on the same team, and high levels of teammate social influence increased odds of clinically significant weight loss by 20 percent. Team captains lost more weight than team members, so feeling responsible for motivating and encouraging their team members may have increased their own motivation. So if you decide to start a trend in your family and friends, you can improve your own health and weight by making healthy, active choices. Tell your friends and family, and encourage them to join you. The social network and support will help everyone achieve better outcomes.

There is a big caveat with regard to your social network and your weight-loss outcomes. If you are the first to lose weight, or if your weight loss may change the social order, friends and family may unconsciously sabotage your weight-loss efforts. You may even unconsciously sabotage your own efforts to get things back to normal. Years ago, I knew a woman who was very obese, and very popular and beloved by all her friends. She didn't drive, and her friends regularly offered their husbands to take her on errands. She lost a lot of weight, and as she did she became more attractive. She noted one day that her friends no longer volunteered their husbands. She actually stated that she had decided that she preferred having friends to being thin, and she went back to her prior eating habits.

This is not an unusual story. In one large survey of 24,000 overweight women, they reported that losing weight created problems in their relationships that regaining the weight resolved. It's not that your friends don't want you to be happy, but they are scared of change, or scared of feeling guilty about their own decisions, or they don't really understand what you're doing, or they just miss how things used to be. If your friends and family are sabotaging your healthy efforts, they probably don't even realize they're doing it. And even if they wanted to help, they might not know how to help, or might have their own beliefs that make it hard for them to understand what you're doing.

At the Duke University Diet and Fitness Center, after a three-week inpatient program, participants write a "Dear supporter" letter to take home to friends and family, which communicates the help that you need. So think about what you really need, and then express that to your friends and family. They can't read your mind. You need to clarify how you need help. Maybe you need to keep a certain food out of the house, because it's a trigger for you to overeat. Maybe you need to eat dinner earlier in the evening. But first, you need to figure out what you need, to support your health, weight, and fitness, and then you need to voice those needs to the ones you love, so that they can support you in the way that you need.

It can be challenging to make a conscious decision in the right direction, because there are unconscious clues in the environment that affect our eating decisions. Research shows that we think that we are all independent individuals capable of making good decisions, especially in light of information. For instance, imagine that you see a picture of a friend on a recent vacation. Your friend is about 25 pounds overweight. As you are looking at the pictures, someone in your office offers you cookies. Will your friend's picture have an impact on how many cookies you eat?

Most people say yes it will, that seeing a picture of an overweight friend will remind them to eat fewer cookies, and 31 percent of people say it will remind them to completely abstain from the cookies. But experimental studies show we're not as good at understanding unconscious motivation as we think we are. In one study, individuals walking through a lobby were randomly stopped and asked to complete a survey. The surveys had photographs of an overweight individual, a normal weight individual, and a lamp. After completing the survey, subjects were told they could help themselves to a bowl of candy. Subjects who were exposed to the picture of the overweight individual took on average 30 percent more candy! In a follow-up study, participants were invited to a cookie taste test. Again, some subjects viewed pictures of an overweight individual, and others viewed pictures of trees, fishbowls, or normal-weight people. Participants who looked at pictures of overweight individuals ate twice as many cookies.

So it may be that seeing people who are overweight unconsciously makes us eat more. But it's even more complicated because social influence also holds up when we eat with other people. Research holds that when we eat with others, we match our portion size to the social norms. So we may eat more or less than we normally eat, based on what the others are eating.

One very interesting study used different types of food, candy and granola, to compare unhealthy versus healthy food. They had a confederate, which is a researcher who pretended to be another study participant, and they had her in two different weight conditions. In her normal condition, she was thin, and they used a prosthetic to make her appear overweight in some of the studies. The interaction provided interesting nuances. When left alone to choose how much food they want, people took and ate almost identical portions of chocolate candy or granola. They took the least amount of food when they watched a thin person take a small portion—about half of what they took when by themselves. When they watched an obese person take a small portion, they took less than they would have by themselves, but more than she took. When they watched an obese person take a large portion, they both took and ate a little more than when they were by themselves. But when they watched a thin person take a large portion, they ate more, and when it was chocolate candy, they ate three times as much!

Eating with people who make good portion-size decisions can influence us to eat less, and when the people who make good portion-size decisions are thin, we will eat less than if the person making a good decision is overweight. Eating with an obese person who eats a large portion will cause us to eat more than we would have on our own. But eating with thin people who eat large portions can actually be the worst influence on our portion-size decisions!

Perhaps we unconsciously think that it must be OK to eat so much, because they are doing it and they are thin, so we follow along. In fact, when researchers assess the impacts of social norms on portion size, they suggest that if you tend to eat small portions you should eat your meals by yourself, because the social norms in group eating may cause you to choose larger portions. In contrast, if you tend to overeat, then you should eat your meals with others, because the social norms may help you to anchor your portion size at a smaller amount, and you will eat less.

Social norms are powerful forms of social control over human behavior. What the people around us do affects what we will do. Research finds that this holds for eating and physical activity behaviors, so if the people we associate go for walks or drink lots of soda or eat lots of fruits and vegetables, we are more likely to do those things, too. So the key, then, is to figure out how to use your social environment to support health-promoting behaviors. For instance, 90 percent of exercise program participants prefer to exercise with a partner or group than to exercise alone. Self-determination theory, which we'll discuss more in Lecture 12, holds that one of the primary motivators for human behavior is connectedness. If you establish a fitness program that helps you feel connected to others, you are more likely to stick with it.

There are multiple variables at play. First, if your fitness program helps foster your sense of connection, then you're getting multiple benefits. You feel better, you get physical health benefits, and it supports your relationship. Second, the sense of commitment to another person may keep you going even when your own motivation lags: If you know your friend is going to be waiting for you at the park to go for a hike, you're more likely to go and less likely to talk yourself out of it. In a couple of research studies I did focused on older adult fitness, I found that the relationships with their classmates and with the instructor were one of the primary motivators that kept people coming to class.

This holds true in families, as well. Pediatricians and child therapists approach a child's obesity as a family problem, not the child's problem. If an obese child is put on a diet and exercise program, it may call attention to the child, increasing feelings of psychological insecurity and actually leading to additional weight gain. But if the whole family makes lifestyle changes, improves their diet, and increases their exercise, it can improve the health and weight for the child in a supportive environment. Research studies have found that maternal and paternal exercise levels can predict a child's activity level. This is also true for changes in a parent's exercise levels, so if a previously inactive and overweight parent becomes more active, the child will, too.

Likewise, though marriage is often shown to increase health and promote longevity, the impact of marriage may depend on the health of your spouse.

If your spouse has poor health, you are more likely to smoke cigarettes and less likely to exercise. In contrast, if you are married and join a fitness program by yourself, the likelihood that you will drop out is 43 percent, but if you join with your spouse, the likelihood you will drop out is only 6.3 percent!

In a study of older adults aged 70–79, married men reported higher levels of exercise, and married women reported higher levels of total activity, non-exercise activity, and exercise. Highly active men were almost three times as likely to have a highly active spouse. So as we get older, our family influence can be particularly strong. I'd encourage you to look at how you can connect with your family, through fitness.

So again back to our centenarians, we know that the people who live the longest exercise and have good social relationships. We know that being lonely or having limited relationships can actually reduce our health. We know that our relationships affect the decisions we make about fitness and exercise. But here's one of the challenges of modern life: Just as we understand how important our social networks are, we find ourselves more isolated. From 1985 to 2004, the mean number of people with whom Americans say they can discuss matters important to them dropped from 2.94 to 2.08, which means that most people went from having three good friends to only two good friends. The number of people who say they have no one to discuss important things with more than doubled in the same two decades, up to 25 percent. For most Americans, the only people they talk to about important matters are family: 80 percent reported in 2004 that all of their confidants were family members.

Researchers have different theories about why our social networks are becoming smaller, and more fragile. People move more, which breaks up the social networks which we were born into. Many of us work more, which means that more of our waking hours are spent either at work or at home. For instance, among college-educated, dual-working couples with children, women work on average 39 hours a week outside the home, plus an additional 32 hours per week of housework, childcare, and errands. Men work 45 hours per week plus an additional 21 hours of housework, childcare, and other household tasks. That's just over 10 hours a day for women, and just under 10 hours a day for men, seven days a week, of work and chores.

On top of that, a Harvard Business School study found that American managers and professionals spent another 40– 50 hours per week still monitoring work on their mobile devices. So even when we're not technically working, we're still in work mindset. No wonder, then, that from 1985 to 2005, leisure time decreased for women, and for men with college educations. In contrast, during the same period, leisure time actually increased for men without a college education. Economists have called it called "leisure inequality," the notion that if you are more educated and better paid, you have less time to enjoy the money you earn.

So look at your own life: You have a schedule packed with paid work, caretaking of kids or parents, plus household chores, and many of your waking hours away from work, you're still on an electronic leash. Add some necessities like sleep and showering and eating, and you'll find you don't have much time left for social interactions. What time you have, you're probably spending online. Survey results show that the average American spends 2 hours a day on social networking, and that those who regularly use social networking sites spend 3.8 hours a day making virtual connections. While those virtual connections can lead to broader social networks, research shows that deeper relationships still require face-to-face interaction. One study found that even for those with broad online social networks, their deep friendships were predominantly formed with face-to-face interactions.

So here is a question for hardworking, mid-career professionals to consider: Do you have any friends outside of work and the Internet? And the really hard follow-up question: Can you really consider your work friends personal friends? Or are they professional colleagues with whom you are friendly? And for your Internet friends, are they real friends, or just avatars?

This is the challenge as we work hard, and plan towards retirement. We are saving money for our retirement years, but are we also taking time to build and nurture the relationships that we will need to have a healthy, happy retirement? If all of your friends are at work, what happens if you lose your job? Or get ill and have to take time off? Will you feel comfortable asking people from work to bring you food and get you to doctor appointments? What happens when you retire: Without the job to discuss, will you still have anything in common? Likewise for your Internet friends: Do they even live in your area? Do you have a relationship that would work in real-time, or is it entirely asynchronous, allowing you to interact without ever really having to make time for each other?

I don't mean to downplay the positive relationships you have at work. They matter, and they make the many hours you spend at the office positive and engaging. Likewise, the social relationships you have online are part of your network. However, I also want to encourage you to think about relationships in the real world and outside of work, and how you can build the kind of social network you need for true fitness and wellness.

It's more difficult to make friends as we get older: People have obligations and requirements that make "hanging out" and building relationships challenging. There are jobs and kids and family needs, things that are urgent. You have to be as deliberate about cultivating relationships as you are about cultivating other aspects of your health and wellness. You need to think about how to support yourself in having opportunities to connect with people. Think about activities you enjoy, causes you believe in, places that you like to be, and fill your life with those things, so that you have the opportunity to connect with people in the places and spaces that make you feel good.

If you'd like to grow old where you are, you should also consider the friendships and relationships around you. As we discussed in our first lecture, most of us outlive our ability to drive. So the people who live around you, the people who live within walking distance, and the people who can drive to you, will become increasingly important in your social environment as you get older. Think deliberately about how to nurture the relationships that are in your neighborhood.

Relationships and social norms have a powerful impact on our health and fitness. Let's think about how you can put that power to good use. When you spend time with your parents, can you get them out for a walk? If they don't walk well, lend an arm for balance; get them outside in the fresh air and sunshine. For date night with your spouse, can you trade in dinner and a movie for a dance class or a partner yoga class? When your kids want to play with can you get active? Hopscotch or jump rope or tag with the little ones, a game of catch or basketball with the older ones.

Perhaps your whole family can take the dog out for a walk around the block after dinner. Maybe your kids or grandkids love videogames; surprise them with an active gaming session, and take them on in a virtual game of tennis or a dance marathon. If you don't have kids or grandkids, volunteer with youth who need you in the area—take a kid who doesn't know anything about botany for a walk through a botanical garden. Maybe meet friends for a golf game, plan a girlfriend getaway at a spa, take a family vacation to a national park.

The point is, think about how you can build your relationships through fitness, how you can get fit through your relationships. You may find it has other positive impacts on your relationships. For instance, maybe your teenage or adult son is a little reluctant to talk about his love life, but loosened up at a batting cage, or side by side while trying out rock-climbing, he may feel more like talking and share some insights with you.

For the takeaway for this lecture, I'd like you to think about how you can better leverage your social network to support your health and well-being. First, assess what kind of social network you have. Do you have friends outside of work, or has your world narrowed to your career? Do you feel like you have a social support system? Do you have anyone who can bring you soup when you're sick, or drive you home from outpatient surgery?

Next, assess the support of your friends and family. Do you have friends and family who could be considered health promoters? If so, how can you better connect with them and ask for their support? Do you have friends who may be unconsciously sabotaging your health and well-being? If so, what can you say to them to help them understand why you are making these changes? How can you help reduce their sense of being threatened? How can you adapt the relationship to improve the friendship while you are improving your health?

In our next lecture, we'll talk about the dark side of fitness, and what happens when promoting exercise and fitness take over your life. Having a balanced sense of wellness, with a strong social network, can help protect you from the obsessive behaviors that may make exercise unhealthy.

Also think about other opportunities you could seek out to build your social relationships. If you loved team sports as a child, maybe you would enjoy a recreational team like volleyball or softball. If you miss playing with your kids when they were little, and you don't have grandkids or they live far away, again, can you volunteer, go to a local school or community center? If you're trying to strengthen your relationship with your parents, can you try a Tai Chi or chair yoga class together? Is there something you have always wanted to learn, or a craft in which you've wanted to try to increase your skills? Try to leverage that into a way of connecting with people who have similar interests. A gardening club, a book club, a line-dance class, maybe a sewing workshop at a community center? Perhaps you have a skill that you can share with others; maybe you can volunteer at a women's shelter, helping young women build their resumes, learning how to interview to get a job. Maybe you can teach knitting, quilting, or cake decorating.

If you're dealing with a health condition, or serving as a caretaker for a loved one, perhaps a targeted support group is a way for you to build connections with people who understand what you are going through. The point overall of the activity though is for you to think about, what are the ways that you could provide yourself opportunities to build new relationships? What are the new ways that you can connect the ones you love with the healthy lifestyle you are working to build? Think about strategies you could try that will help you build new friendships, and strengthen the relationships you have.

The bottom line is that whether you are aware of it or not, whether you want them to or not, your friends and family are going to impact the food you eat, the exercise you do, and the size of your waistline. You can choose to be more conscious and more aware, to put that social influence to good use for you, and for your loved ones.

Accepting a New Reality
Lecture 9

A plan for healthy aging requires you to be deliberate about exercise and healthy eating, but the point is to exercise and eat healthfully so that you are healthy enough to live a full, engaging life. When fitness and exercise become your central focus—when you live to exercise and eat healthfully—then you are no longer aging healthfully. If you find that the activities that should promote health are beginning to consume your life, you may have a problem. In this lecture, we will discuss eating disorders, exercise addiction, and overtraining. Our goal is to become aware of the potential pitfalls so that you can keep your life in balance.

Scope and Types of Eating Disorders

- When we think about anorexia, we usually picture an already thin teenage girl starving herself, and it's true that anorexia overwhelmingly occurs among adolescent girls. But from 2001 to 2010, the rate of eating disorders among middle-aged adults increased by 42%. A study of adults between the ages of 55 and 64 showed similar increases.

  - By official counts, at least 11% of older women—more than 1 in 10—suffer from an eating disorder.

  - Far more have subclinical problems with body dissatisfaction and live their lives structured around diet and exercise. In a 2010 study by the Oregon Health and Science University, women between the ages of 65 and 80 were just as likely as young adult women to express concerns about body shape or indicate that they felt fat.

- Bulimia is the combination of binging and purging. An individual with bulimia may consume a large amount of food in a short time and then compensate by purging. Purging can take many forms, including forced vomiting, use of laxatives and/or diuretics, excessive exercise, and fasting. Individuals with bulimia may or may not be underweight.

- o Purging via exercise can be particularly sneaky, because it can start out as a healthy practice. Older men in particular may be prone to compulsive exercise.

- o Bulimia may be hard for others to notice because individuals with bulimia are often at a normal weight or even slightly overweight, rather than excessively thin. No one suspects an eating disorder.

- Individuals who have anorexia severely limit the quantity and often the types of food they eat. These individuals may be extremely thin and are preoccupied with their weight, often seeing themselves as heavier than they are. Older women with anorexia usually are not emaciated and, in fact, may be praised by their doctors for keeping their weight down.

- o Anorexia can be particularly challenging in older adults because health conditions may require an individual to restrict or limit food consumption. For instance, an individual with high cholesterol or type II diabetes should limit consumption of sugars, refined flours, or saturated fat.

- o Such food limitations can start for health-promoting reasons but end up being so extreme that they affect the individual's quality of life. An important consideration is whether or not the individual is maintaining a healthy weight and experiencing overall good health.

- An individual who suffers from a binge-eating disorder regularly eats a large amount of food in a short period of time, usually in secret and often with feelings of guilt or shame. In contrast to individuals with bulimia, individuals with binge-eating disorder don't follow the binge with a purge. They are often overweight or obese; they may even be in denial about how many calories they consume and the source of their weight.

- Eating and body image disorders can also manifest themselves in other ways, such as a preoccupation with plastic surgery. Men with muscle dysmorphia may think that they are too small or skinny, regardless of how much muscle mass they actually have. They may focus as obsessively on getting bigger as women with anorexia focus on getting smaller.

Causes of Eating Disorders

- In a small number of cases, eating disorders occur late in life as the result of a stressor or a medical condition. For instance, if an individual loses weight because of an illness, particularly if she has previously struggled with her weight, she may receive compliments about her new, slender appearance. This can lead to a focus on food restriction after recovery. Medical conditions may also require individuals to go on more restricted diets; they may then become preoccupied with controlling diet as a way of controlling their health.

- In most cases, those who suffer from eating disorders later in life also suffered from them in adolescence. Sometimes, the severity increases in older adults, bringing new and more difficult symptoms. Ninety-four percent of middle-aged women with anorexia had an eating disorder when they were younger.

- Common stressors that may lead to the development or recurrence of an eating disorder include difficulty adjusting to changes in the body and perceived level of attractiveness; the death of a loved one, which can lead to feelings of lack

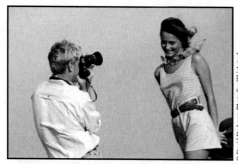

© David De Lossy/Photodisc/Thinkstock.

One study found that most models and actresses are 20% below ideal body weight, yet they strongly influence our perceptions of beauty.

of control; and divorce. Of course, societal pressure to be thin also influences all of us, including older adults.

- o An article in the *Journal of Nutrition for the Elderly* reported that advertising targeted at older adults focuses on anti-aging and health-promoting products and that these advertisements can have a negative impact on body image.

- o In one study of women aged 60 to 70, 45% reported that their self-esteem depended on their weight and shape, and more than 60% reported that they had only moderate or low satisfaction with their weight and shape.

- o If we have unrealistic expectations about how we should look as we age, we may become vulnerable to unhealthy patterns of diet and exercise.

- Sometimes, the disconnect between how we feel and how we look can cause a problem. A 2009 Pew Research Center study found that 60% of people over age 65 feel younger than they are, but the mirror may not reflect the youth they still feel. If you've always been fit and healthy, those changes in the mirror may be particularly hard to take.

- For both new and recurring eating disorders, stressors associated with caretaking can accidentally trigger an eating disorder. Those serving as primary caretakers for a loved one may not have the time to eat or take care of themselves properly; this situation may eventually lead to a formal eating disorder.

Getting Help
- Older adults often struggle with shame when they have an eating disorder. They believe that they should know better or be able to overcome the disorder on their own. This shame can make treatment challenging. Many treatment centers now separate patients over and under 30 to make adults feel more comfortable talking about the unique issues of eating disorders in adulthood.

- If you have any concerns about your own eating behaviors or those of a loved one, it's important to find a therapist or center that has experience working with older adults in a setting that is respectful of life experience and age.

- Treatment often includes cognitive behavioral therapy, which will help address unrealistic thoughts about food and appearance. Treatment may also include work with a dietician or nutritional counselor to help individuals learn or relearn the components of a healthy diet and address nutritional imbalances brought about by disordered eating.

Exercise Addiction

- Exercise addiction is a psychological or physiological dependence on a regular regimen of exercise that is characterized by withdrawal symptoms after 24 to 36 hours without exercise. It typically includes both psychological and physiological factors.

- In contrast to a healthy commitment to exercise, exercise addiction leads individuals to structure their lives around fitness. They may continue to exercise even when injured or at the expense of other obligations. When an exercise-addicted person can't exercise, he or she may feel withdrawal symptoms, such as anxiety, muscle twitching, and irritability.

- Exercise addiction may be connected to a specific form of exercise that the individual views as best promoting health and fitness. It may be more likely to occur with solitary fitness activities, such as running, biking, and swimming. Moving to more social forms of fitness can help overcome the isolating effects of exercise addiction.

- Some researchers believe that exercise addiction is related to brain chemistry. Studies have shown, for example, that extreme exercise in rats changes their levels of dopamine, a neurotransmitter that is related to mood in both rats and humans.

167

- Researchers estimate that exercise addiction occurs in about 3% of the general population, but one study of regular participants at a fitness club found that 42% of the individuals at the club met the criteria for exercise addiction. It is also likely to co-occur with an eating disorder; as many as 48% of individuals with an eating disorder also meet the criteria for exercise addiction.

Overtraining

- Overtraining occurs when an individual trains beyond the body's capacity to rest and recover, which may lead to such symptoms as fatigue, achy muscles, joint pain, insomnia, headaches, and more.

- Research shows that regular exercise boosts the immune system, but high-intensity or excessive exercise may actually decrease immunity. One study found that 90 minutes of high-intensity exercise can make you more susceptible to illness for 72 hours after the exercise. Other research shows that endurance athletes are at increased risk for upper respiratory tract infections, both during heavy training and during the 1 to 2 weeks after racing.

- To prevent overtraining, you need to be realistic in setting your goals to prevent injury and allot sufficient time for rest and recovery. In addition, the goals you set now may need to be modified as you get older or if you experience an illness or injury.

Realistic Expectations

- Even if you're not suffering from an eating disorder, the physical changes of aging can lower your confidence and self-esteem. If there are aspects of your appearance that you've always identified as an important part of you, it can be hard to figure out who you are as your appearance changes. If you've worked hard to keep your body trim and in shape, you may notice with frustration that your face shows more age than the faces of your plumper peers.

- To combat negative feelings, think about what really matters to you. It's fine to have goals related to your appearance, but make sure they are realistic and attainable. Focus on looking the best you can now so that you can enjoy who you are and how you look.

- Remember that your fitness activities should support and improve your life. Your life should not be exclusively about supporting and improving your fitness activities. The goal isn't fitness for the sake of fitness but fitness that supports holistic well-being.

Suggested Reading

Maine, *The Body Myth*.

Powers and Thompson, *The Exercise Balance*.

Activities and Assignments

Find a quiet place to do some honest soul-searching. In your journal, reflect on the following questions: Are you doing anything in the pursuit of healthiness that has become unhealthy? Do you have any current beliefs about your fitness, your looks, or your body that are affecting your sense of self-esteem and wellness? Think through what you believe, feel, or are currently doing that is promoting dysfunction instead of wellness and brainstorm how you could do something different, new, or creative to promote wellness.

Take your journal with you to a mirror in a well-lit room, preferably with natural light. Look at yourself in the mirror. Write in your journal at least five things that you like about your body (strengths, abilities, and so on) and five things that you like about your appearance. Use the nonjudgmental framework we discussed in our lecture on mindfulness; look at yourself with loving kindness. If you find that negative, critical, or judgmental thoughts wander in, push them aside and let them go.

Accepting a New Reality

Lecture 9—Transcript

When we talk about fitness for healthy aging, what we're talking about is how to grow to accept a new reality. And that means everything in moderation—including fitness and healthy eating. A plan for healthy aging requires you to be deliberate about exercise and your diet. But the point is to exercise and eat healthfully so that you are healthy enough to live a full, engaging life. There can be a dark side. When fitness and exercise become your central focus—when you are suddenly living to exercise and eat healthfully—then you are no longer aging healthfully. If you find that the activities that should promote health are beginning to consume your life, you may have a problem.

In this lecture, we will discuss eating disorders, exercise addiction, and overtraining. Our goal for this lecture is to help you become aware of the potential pitfalls, so that you can keep your life in balance, and keep your exercise and diet as the healthy foundation to a full, enriched life.

If you think about death by anorexia, you probably picture an already-thin teenage girl starving herself into an early grave. And it's true that anorexia overwhelmingly occurs among adolescent girls. Of those girls, 5–10 percent will die within 10 years. Only about 1 in 10 will receive treatment, and only 30–40 percent will actually recover. Most of the rest will suffer their entire lives with low self-esteem and disordered eating and still die prematurely; in fact, the average age of death for a woman with anorexia is 69 years old. In contrast, the average life expectancy of a woman in the U.S. is 85.

From 2001 to 2010, the rate of eating disorders among middle-aged adults increased by 42 percent. A study of adults between the ages of 55 and 64 showed similar increases: Binge eating increased from 1.7 percent of individuals in 1995 to 7.4 percent in 2005, and strict dieting or fasting went from 0 percent in 1995 to 9.7 percent in 2005. More than half of the patients at the Eating Disorders Program at the University of North Carolina are adults, not teenagers. The Renfrew Center, which is the largest network of eating disorder clinics in the U.S., saw a 42-percent increase in patients over the age of 35, and has specifically added a treatment track for midlife adults.

Eight percent of women over the age of 50 suffer from bulimia, which is binging and then purging, either through vomiting, laxatives, or excessive exercise. Men may do it too; men in professions that impose weight or appearance requirements such as the military or other uniformed professions may be at risk as they get older and find it harder to meet their weight limits. Some of these men may find themselves using laxatives and diuretics to lose weight before a weigh-in.

Eating disorders like bulimia and anorexia most often occur in white women, but binge eating does not discriminate by race. According to research, equal numbers of white, black, and Hispanic women are affected: 3.5 percent of women older than 50 have binge eating disorder, and 2.5 percent of adult men meet the clinical criteria for binge eating disorder. Binge eating isn't just overeating at a party; it's when eating interferes with work, family, and social life, and when the individual feels that eating has become unmanageable. The individual ends up feeling a sense of despair and disgust, and feeling like they've lost control.

So official counts hold that at least 11 percent of older women, more than 1 in 10, are suffering from an eating disorder. Far more have sub-clinical problems with body dissatisfaction, and live their lives structured around diet and exercise. A 2012 study in the *International Journal of Eating Disorders* reported that 13 percent of women over the age of 50 exhibit eating disorder symptoms. For a sense of scale, 12 percent of women in the same age group have breast cancer. In at 2010 study by the Oregon Health & Science University, women between the ages of 65 to 80 were just as likely as young adult women to express concerns about body shape or indicate that they feel fat. This is a larger problem for older adults than we realize or like to talk about.

Let's talk about the types of eating disorders in particular. Bulimia: the combination of binging and purging. An individual with bulimia may consume a large amount of food in a short time and then compensate by purging. Purging can take many forms, as we said: forced vomiting, use of laxatives or diuretics, excessive exercise, even fasting. Individuals with bulimia may or may not be underweight; often, they have normal body weights. The purging can be in the form of deals you make with yourself: I want to eat this big dinner, so I'll eat salad all next week. I want to have ice cream tonight at the party, so I won't eat anything tomorrow. I'm going out tonight, so I won't eat anything today.

Purging via exercise can be particularly sneaky. It starts out healthy, and doesn't seem like a problem. You go out for a run the morning after you ate too much at a party—that's probably not a problem, that's probably just burning off the calories. But what if you start doing it every weekend? What if you start doing it a couple of times a week? What happens when you start making deals with yourself: I can eat this cake and have this drink, if I run on the treadmill for an hour tomorrow? I can eat this bag of spicy chips and cheese, and I'll take two hot yoga classes tomorrow to sweat it out. Older men in particular may be prone to compulsive exercise. Bulimia can also be hard for others to notice, because as we said individuals with bulimia are often normal weight; sometimes they're slightly overweight, rather than excessively thin. So no one suspects an eating disorder.

Anorexia is the severe restriction of eating. Individuals with anorexia limit the quantity, and often the types, of food they eat. Individuals with anorexia may be extremely thin, and are often preoccupied with their weight, seeing themselves as heavier than they are. Older women with anorexia usually are not emaciated, and in fact may be praised by their doctors for keeping their weight down. In young women, the loss of the menses is a classic sign of anorexia, but that is not a helpful to diagnose anorexia in older women who may have already gone through menopause.

Anorexia can be particularly challenging in older adults, because health conditions may require an individual to restrict or limit food consumption. For instance, for an individual with high cholesterol or type-2 diabetes, it may be appropriate to limit consumption of sugars, refined flours, and saturated fat. Food limitations can start out for health-promoting reasons, but then they end up so extreme that they damage quality of life. An important consideration is, how are those dietary restrictions are impacting the individual's quality of life? Is the individual maintaining a healthy weight and are they experiencing overall good health.?

I have been a vegetarian since I was 17. Among vegetarian friends, I have seen a wide range of healthy to unhealthy behaviors. I know individuals who are raw foodists or vegans and who have strict limitations in their diets, but they're deliberate to eat healthy, to eat health-promoting foods, to eat appropriate quantities, and so they have good health and maintain a healthy weight and an active lifestyle. In contrast, I have known some individuals who use strict forms of vegetarianism as a way to make dieting easy, and to maintain low weight, low body fat, and they suffer ill health as a result. So the bottom line on what is healthy eating is the outcome: What is the person's overall health and overall quality of life?

Binge eating disorder, again when an individual regularly eats a large amount of food in a short period of time. Binge eating is usually done in secret, and often related to feelings of guilt or shame. In contrast to individuals with bulimia, who also binge, individuals with binge eating disorder don't follow the binge with a purge. They are often overweight or obese. In many cases, they may eat appropriate or healthy portion sizes when they are around other individuals, and binge in secret; often the binging is related to coping with stress or numbing their feelings. Because what's called a double-life for binge eaters, they may even be in denial about how many calories they are consuming and the source of their weight, saying "I don't understand why I'm overweight. I eat a normal amount" because they have a hard time accepting the binges that occur.

Years ago, as an example, I knew a woman who weighed over 300 pounds. She ate normal portion sizes during the day at work. But on the way home from work, in the midst of stress and frustration, she would stop at a gas station and buy an extra-large soda (full sugar, not diet), a bag of candy, and a full-size bag of potato chips. She would discover that she'd eaten all of it before she got home. She'd try to be healthy; she'd make a healthy dinner, with an appropriate-sized portion of vegetables, whole grains, and proteins. But after dinner, she'd be watching television, she would find herself on her couch, full gallon container of ice cream empty. She felt embarrassed and out of control about her eating, and struggled to admit it to herself. When she began addressing other areas of her life where she felt out of control (her finances, the organization of her work life, her home, her personal life) she started to feel more in control of her life, and she began to feel more in control of her eating, and that was when she was able to gain control of her binges.

Eating and body image disorders can also manifest themselves in other ways, for instance, a preoccupation with plastic surgery. Some individuals even completely avoid looking at themselves in the mirror, a practice some psychologists have termed "mirror fasting." Men with muscle dysmorphia may always think they are too small, too scrawny, regardless of how much muscle mass they actually have. They may focus as obsessively on getting bigger as women with anorexia focus on getting smaller.

We've talked a lot up until this point in the course about how to promote a healthier attitude toward food and exercise, how to build calorie burning into your life more regularly, and make better choices that promote your health. But when calories, whether consumed or burned, become the center of your life, that's when you have a problem. When food and exercise are no longer about helping you be healthy, to live a full, happy life, but instead become the central focus of who you are, that's an indication that something is out of balance.

So what happens to create that imbalance? In a small number of cases, it occurs late in life due to a stressor or another medical condition. For instance, if an individual loses weight due to an illness, particularly if she has previously struggled with her weight, she may actually receive compliments about her new slender appearance. This can lead to a new focus on food restriction after recovery from the illness. A medical condition can require an individual to go on a restricted diet, such as a heart attack or stroke—doctors may restrict certain foods during recovery. The individual may become preoccupied with controlling his diet as a way of controlling his health.

Most cases, though, are either individuals who developed eating disorders in adolescence and suffered their entire lives, or who suffered, recovered, and then experienced a recurrence later in life, often due to a significant change or stressor. In some cases, the severity increases in the older adult, bringing new and more difficult symptoms. For middle-aged women with anorexia in particular, there appears to be a history of prior eating problems: 94 percent experienced an eating disorder when they were younger.

There are common stressors that may lead to the development or recurrence of an eating disorder. For instance, difficulty adjusting to changes in your body and perceived level of attractiveness after having children or going through menopause may be a stressor for many women. For both men and women, the death of a loved one can lead to feelings of lack of control, and eating and exercise become something that you feel like you can control. Likewise, the sense of loss that occurs in divorce can leave individuals feeling unloved and unattractive, leading to an obsessive focus on appearance and controlling that aspect of the self. Obsessive behaviors can occur as a reaction in an attempt to regain a sense of control. Loss in particular may be a powerful trigger for the development or resurgence of an eating disorder.

There are also societal pressures which influence all of us. Every day, we see actors and models who have had their photographs digitally manipulated into unrealistic portrayals of attractiveness. One research study found that most models and actresses on television are 20 percent below ideal body weight. Twenty percent below ideal body weight means they meet one of the criteria for anorexia, but they influence what as a culture we think beautiful women looks like. Actors and models, men and women, of all ages are Photoshopped into perfection, blemishes wrinkles, everything wiped away, so that we have unrealistic expectations of what beauty looks like.

To get a dose of reality, log onto the Internet and look for images of celebrities before and after they've been altered. You'll be amazed at what attractive really looks like, versus what the media thinks it should look like. They tuck waists, trim hips, smooth lines, and brighten skin tone, make arms skinnier, all sorts of things the media does to attractive men and women regardless of their age, to make them even more attractive, which just makes it harder for the rest of us how we look in real life. An article in the *Journal of Nutrition for the Elderly* reported that advertising targeted at older adults focuses on anti-aging and health-promoting products, and that article concluded that these advertisements can have negative body image impacts.

One study of women aged 60 to 70 found that 45 percent of those women reported that their self-esteem depended on their weight and shape, and over 60 percent of them reported that they had only moderate or low satisfaction with their weight and shape. If we have these unrealistic expectations about how we should look as we age, it can make us vulnerable to unhealthy patterns of diet and exercise in an attempt to achieve something that we think we should have.

Sometimes, it's also our own disconnect between how we feel and how we look that can cause a problem. A 2009 Pew Research Center study found that 60 percent of people over the age of 65 feel younger than they are, and almost half feel at least 10 years younger than their actual age, but when you look in the mirror it might not reflect the youth you still feel. If you've always been fit and healthy and in shape, changes in the mirror can be particularly hard to take, and we have to adjust to that as part of accepting a new healthy reality as we get older.

Sometimes, for both new and recurring eating disorders, stressors associated with caretaking can trigger an issue. For instance, if you're serving as a primary caretaker for a loved one, you may not have the time to eat—you're rushing about, you're stressed, you're not taking care of yourself. This could eventually lead to the manifestation of a problematic behavior, especially if you've had a prior issue that could recur.

Shame is an emotion that older adults who have an eating disorder struggle with. Individuals in treatment express feeling like they should know better, they should have overcome it, they should be able to be a role model to the people younger than them. This shame makes it hard to talk about, and that can make treatment challenging. In fact, some eating disorder treatment centers have found that if older adults are in therapy sessions with younger adults, the older adults often remain silent and don't participate. Many treatment centers now separate people over and under the age of 30, to make adults feel more comfortable talking about the unique issues of eating disorders in adulthood.

It's important to get help, because the impacts of eating disorders when untreated can be profound. They can make bone density loss worse, which quickens the pace of osteoporosis and makes injuries from falls more likely. They can lead to tooth erosion. They can damage the gastrointestinal system; they can damage the heart. If you have any concerns about your own eating behaviors, or the eating behaviors of a loved one, it's important to work with a therapist or center that has experience working with older adults, and in a setting that is respectful of your life experience and age.

Treatment will include psychotherapy, in particular, cognitive behavioral therapy, which will help address the unrealistic thoughts about food and appearance and help you develop healthier and more supportive patterns. You should work with a dietician or nutritional counselor to help you learn or relearn the components of a healthy diet and also address any nutritional imbalances brought about by disordered eating. Whether you're dealing with a new issue, the recurrence of an old wound, or you've been struggling for decades, you can recover. In fact, research shows that middle-aged and older adults in treatment for eating disorders are often more determined and more ready to recover.

If your fitness lifestyle takes over and fitness become the problem, you may be experiencing exercise addiction. Exercise addiction is a psychological or physiological dependence on a regular regimen of exercise that is characterized by withdrawal symptoms after 24 to 36 hours without exercise. It typically includes both psychological and physiological factors.

Let's compare an exercise addiction to a healthy commitment to exercise. When you have a healthy commitment to exercise, you have developed a habit of daily activity, and your regular exercise produces psychological benefits and supports your well-being and functioning. However, for some people, this healthy habit can begin to control their lives. When exercise addiction occurs, the individual believes he or she has to structure their life around their fitness. This belief eliminates other choices, and this person may continue to exercise even when they are injured or when their social and occupational needs should come first. When an exercise-addicted person can't exercise, he or she may feel withdrawal symptoms, such as anxiety, muscle twitching, irritability, guilt, bloatedness, feelings of nervousness, anger, and depression.

Often exercise addiction may be connected to a specific form of exercise that the individual views as best for promoting their health and fitness. Other forms of exercise won't eliminate or alleviate the withdrawal symptoms. For instance, an injured runner may swim or ride a bike and still not feel like they're getting a good workout. This is also a way that exercise addiction is different from exercise commitment: When you're committed to fitness, you understand cognitively that different types of exercise provide benefits. When you're addicted to exercise, you may think that different types of exercise don't actually count as your workout.

Exercise addiction may be more likely to occur with solitary fitness activities, so running, biking, and swimming, things that you can do on your own. Moving to more social forms of fitness can help overcome the isolating effects of exercise addiction. Some researchers think that exercise addiction is related to neurotransmitters. This line of research has found that even rats may be susceptible to exercise addiction. When rats are exposed to extreme exercise, it actually changes their levels of the neurotransmitter dopamine, which is related to mood in both rats and humans!

The prevalence of exercise addiction varies. Researchers estimate it occurs in about 3 percent of the general population, but one study of regular participants at a fitness club found that 42 percent of the individuals at the club met the criteria for exercise addiction. And it is likely to co-occur with an eating disorder: As many as 48 percent of individuals with an eating disorder also meet the criteria for exercise addiction.

You need to stay fit, but you also need to stay flexible and adaptive. You need to be able to take a day off if circumstances dictate. You also need to be able to recognize other forms of exercise as counting for your workout. If you go for a 10-mile hike with your son or grandson's Boy Scout troop, you probably don't need to go for a separate run. If you spend the afternoon at the pool swimming with friends, being active in the water, maybe you don't need to go to the gym that day. If you help a friend move furniture all afternoon, you probably don't need to lift weights that day for strength training. Remember that activity comes in many forms, and a healthy lifestyle requires a balanced approach to fitness.

Think about how your body feels, both after the exercise, and when you wake up in the morning. If you're exercising so hard that you're waking up tired and in pain every day, you may be exercising too much, or too hard. If you keep pushing and training harder, without sufficient time to rest and recover, it can lead to overtraining. Overtraining occurs when you train beyond your body's capacity to rest and recover. Without sufficient rest and recovery time, you can experience a decline in health. Symptoms include feeling tired and drained, achy muscles, pain in your joints, insomnia and headaches, moodiness, loss of enthusiasm, increased risk for injuries, and even decreased immunity.

We're back to the everything in moderation principle. For instance, research shows that regular exercise boosts the immune system. Moderate exercise is linked to a positive immune response. Immune cells actually become more able to kill bacteria and viruses in people who exercise regularly. One study of the cumulative effects of exercise found that people who walk for 40 minutes per day had half as many sick days due to colds or sore throats than people who don't exercise. However, research also shows that high-intensity or excessive exercise may decrease your immunity. One study found that 90 minutes of high-intensity exercise can make you more susceptible to illness for 72 hours after the exercise. Other research shows that endurance athletes are at increased risk for upper respiratory tract infections both during heavy training and during the 1–2 weeks after racing. Marathon runners are at a higher risk than normal for developing melanoma, which may be related both to the fact that they spend a lot of time running outside, in the sun, and also due to the immune-suppressing effects of ongoing, high-intensity training.

To prevent overtraining, you need to be realistic in setting your training goals to prevent injury, and allot sufficient time for rest and recovery in your training plan. Consider that the goals you set now may have to be modified as you get older, or if you experience an illness or an injury. This is not failure; this is being aware of and responsible to where you are at a particular point in your life.

Think critically about how much pain is necessary versus how much pain is too much. Overcome the "no pain, no gain" mentality. When you are older, your body takes longer to heal from injuries, and you need to take a long-view approach in training. Build in rest periods. Be deliberate about self-care. If you're training for a big event like a marathon, make time to get massages and help your muscles heal. Use ice and heat appropriately to reduce swelling and help you deal with chronic pain. It's also important that you eat and hydrate mindfully to support your body being healthy in your fitness program. For instance, drink your water throughout the day, rather than trying to glug down eight glasses at once, and add additional fluid when it's hot or when you're sweating a great deal.

Even if you're not suffering from an eating disorder or exercise disorder behavior, the physical changes of aging can lower your confidence and your self-esteem. If there are aspects of your appearance that you've always identified as an important part of you, it can be hard to figure out who you are as your appearance changes. A man who has always had a thick, full head of hair, or a woman who has always had long, flowing hair, may find it hard if it age-related thinning starts to make their hair look a little less lush than they're used to. If you've worked hard to keep your body trim and in shape, you may notice with frustration that your face shows more age than plumper peers. French actress Catherine Deneuve has been quoted as saying that there comes an age when you have to choose between your fanny and your face, and that's true for women and men, because the same fat cells that make our bottoms and abdomens bigger than we like also plump up our faces to keep the lines from settling in.

You should also take a good look at your closet. Are your clothes helping you to feel good about yourself, or are they judging you? If you have clothes in your closet that are too small or don't fit well, donate them. Give them to someone else who needs them. It's negative psychological energy to hold on to those wishes for what you should look like. Focus on feeling healthy and well and looking good with what you look like. If you lose weight later, you can reward yourself with new clothes. Be healthy now, in clothes that fit you now. Look at the size, the style, the cut, look for clothes that flatter your shape. If you need help figuring out what that best look or cut is, visit a personal shopper at a department store. You might be amazed at how small decisions can affect so dramatically how something looks on you to make you feel better about yourself.

Watch a few old movies to get a sense of how really small details can make a look. If you watch *An American in Paris* and look at Gene Kelly, look at his fitted polo shirts and how they were specifically designed to emphasize his muscular physique and make his dancing look masculine. Try watching a a Cary Grant movie and notice how his suits, his shirts fit perfectly—he literally had his sleeves tailored to specifications of an eighth of an inch. Think about how you can use your clothes to help you look your best, and get rid of anything that doesn't make you feel great. Don't allow your closet to be a punitive psychological space that just makes you feel worse about yourself.

Overall, think about what really matters to you. It's OK for looking good to be part of your goals; you just need to set your appearance goals in a context that is realistic and attainable. Focus on looking the best you can now, for who you are now, so that you can enjoy who you are and how you look. Go back to Lecture 7, where we talked about goal setting, and think about some SMART goals that you can set that will help you feel good about yourself when you look in the mirror.

Remember above all that your fitness activities should support and improve your life. Your life should not be exclusively about supporting and improving your fitness activities. I completed one of my yoga instructor certifications with David Swenson, a master yoga teacher. During a question and answer part of the course, all the students were asking how do we integrate yoga and other forms of fitness. So people asked, will yoga help me ride my bike, will it help me climb mountains, and David discussed how yoga could help with all of those activities. Then people asked, will riding my bike or climbing mountains make me worse at yoga? He answered that yoga makes you better at everything you do, but everything else you do reduces your "perfection" in yoga. If you climb mountains or ride bikes, it will change your flexibility, and that might make some yoga poses more challenging.

So he said, the key question to ask yourself is why are you doing yoga? Are you doing yoga just to do yoga? In that case, everything you do will interfere. If you're doing yoga to enhance your life, then yoga will improve everything in your life. So ask yourself the same question. Are you doing your fitness and exercise for the sake of exercise? Or to improve the rest of your life? That mindset may shift how you view your fitness program. It's not just fitness for the sake of fitness; it's fitness to support holistic well-being.

As a takeaway activity for this lecture, I'd like you to get out your journal, find a quiet space to think, and do some honest soul-searching. Are you doing anything in the pursuit of healthiness that has become unhealthy? Do you have any current beliefs about your fitness, your looks, or your body that are affecting your sense of self-esteemyou're your overall wellness? Think through what you believe, feel, or are currently doing that could be promoting dysfunction, instead of wellness, and brainstorm how you could do something different, new, or creative to promote wellness.

Next, I'd like you to do another self-reflection exercise, just as difficult. Take your journal with you to a mirror in a well-lit room, preferably with natural light. Look at yourself in the mirror. Write in your journal at least five things that you like about your body in particular, and then write down five things that you like about your overall appearance. Use the non-judgmental framework we discussed in our lecture on mindfulness. Look at yourself with loving kindness. If you find that negative, critical, judgmental thoughts wander in, discard them and let them go. Look for positives. Identify five things you like. These may include strengths, abilities, what you are able to accomplish thanks to your body. For your appearance, think about things you like, like a bright smile, or a crooked nose that reminds you of your mother, a scar from a childhood adventure. They don't have to be things society would think of as beauty, just things that make you who you are, and that make you happy that you are you and that they are part of you. The point is for you to think about the good parts of yourself, to focus on what you like, what is beautiful, and what is strong.

I read a great quote in a magazine that said "at some point, no matter how well you take care of yourself, and how much you exercise, at some point, you're going to have to accept that you look like a healthy, well-rested 40-year-old or 60-year-old or 80-year-old, and you're never going to look 20 again." So let's look toward role models of men and women who age with grace and dignity, instead of those who try to cling to the youth they've lost. Find the beauty and power in the age that you are. We don't have the capacity to regain our youth, but we can maintain our health, and look and feel the best we can, for the age we are.

Challenges—Illness and Chronic Pain
Lecture 10

Y our response to illness, disability, or a chronic health condition plays a large part in determining the quality of the rest of your life. Your ability to maintain or rebuild your physical independence requires you to be motivated to work through physical activity even when it's difficult. Recovering from illness or living with chronic pain calls for a multifaceted approach to self-care, the right medical support, and social support from friends and family. But at the same time that you need to accept help from your loved ones, in the end, you must take responsibility to work through discomforts so that you can rebuild your health and strength.

Chronic Pain

- Acute pain comes on suddenly, is sharp, and usually indicates an injury. This kind of pain occurs when you break a bone, strain a muscle, have dental work or surgery, or have an illness. Acute pain recedes when the underlying condition has been healed.

- Chronic pain occurs through a variety of conditions, such as arthritis, fibromyalgia, or Parkinson's disease. It may be a consequence of complications in advanced diabetes or such illnesses as shingles. As we get older, the body sometimes heals more slowly, and the acute pain of surgery can lead to chronic pain in the surgical area—a shoulder or knee or hip that never feels quite right.

- Chronic pain affects more Americans than diabetes, heart disease, and cancer combined. Approximately 1 in 4 adults experiences chronic pain, with the most common types of chronic pain being low back pain (27%), severe headaches or migraines (15%), neck pain (15%), and facial ache or pain (4%).

- Chronic pain may affect quality of life and life satisfaction more than any other single factor. Sixty percent of chronic pain sufferers say that chronic pain reduces their enjoyment of life, 77% report feelings of depression, and 86% report that pain affects their sleep. The effects of chronic pain can be long lasting. Some studies indicate that the average individual with chronic pain suffers for 7 years and more than 1/5 endure pain for more than 20 years.

- In the United States, we spend more than $635 billion per year on chronic pain. Some of that money goes to pain medicine, including opiates, which can be addictive and can lead to increased sensitivity to pain.

Pain Management
- Physicians specializing in chronic pain recommend a holistic approach to pain management. With chronic pain, treatment focuses on education, social support, and guidance in developing an appropriate program of physical activity and exercise. The goal is to help patients live active lives in spite of the pain they experience.

- Pain is a multidimensional experience with four key aspects: (1) the physiological-sensory dimension—your body's internal response to pain; (2) the affect dimension—your emotional response to pain; (3) the cognitive dimension—your attitudes and beliefs about pain; and (4) the behavioral dimension—the actions you take when pain occurs.

- Research indicates that a multidimensional approach to pain management is the most effective strategy for helping reduce pain and improve function. For instance, when individuals with chronic pain receive education about pain, including its components and psychological strategies for coping, they experience improved attitudes and even reduced pain.
  - Research has found that education programs that focus on understanding and coping strategies may actually be as effective as non-steroidal anti-inflammatories in reducing pain, without the potential side effects of pain medicine.

  - Social support—and education of family members or caregivers—can also be an important part of pain management.

- Physical activity may be one of the most effective treatments for managing chronic pain. Exercise can reduce the experience of chronic pain and improve functional independence. To improve the potential for positive outcomes in pain management via exercise, it's important to have flexible goals that can be adapted based on the level of pain experienced and changes in condition. You also need to pace yourself, be part of the decision-making process about your exercise program, and work with a trained professional who has experience in chronic pain and your specific condition.

- Chronic pain is often accompanied by chronic fatigue, and those who experience chronic pain may feel too tired to exercise. However, research shows that gentle forms of exercise, such as yoga or water aerobics, can improve energy and vigor and reduce pain and fatigue. In fact, inactivity may actually exacerbate the symptoms of chronic pain and fatigue.

- Mindfulness activities can be particularly helpful with chronic pain management. Such fitness practices as yoga and Tai Chi are usually very gentle; thus, you can participate with low risk of injury. These practices also help connect you to awareness of the present moment so that you can learn how to better manage the fear or anxiety associated with pain. Massage and acupuncture are complementary therapies that may also be helpful in coping with chronic pain.

Exercise Options
- If you are in the hospital or restricted to bed, you can still move to keep up your strength and keep yourself active. Moving when and how you can will keep you from putting too much pressure on any one spot of the body, preventing skin ulcers and bedsores. While you're on bed rest, collaborate with the physical and occupational therapists who want to help you get back on your feet as soon as possible.
  - Squeeze gripper balls to maintain your hand strength and do as much as you can for yourself, such as brushing your teeth, feeding yourself, and so on.

- ○ Try gentle stretches of your neck, arms, and shoulders, and if it's safe for you to move your legs, spend a few minutes every hour pointing and flexing your toes. Alternate lifting your legs off the bed.

- ○ Practice focused abdominal breathing to help keep your lungs clear and strong.

- If you're able to sit in a chair or wheelchair, you can do these same exercises and some additional ones. Do upper-body strengthening exercises using hand weights, resistance bands, or even water bottles or soup cans. If you have some use of your legs, you can do leg lifts or stretches with resistance bands. During physical therapy, you may be able to use bicycling or rowing machines to maintain or improve your endurance.

- If you are able to walk with the use of a walker or cane, it's important for you to stay as active as you can to either maintain the walking capacity you have, or, if possible, rebuild your strength for independent walking. You can do both the bed-based activities and chair-based exercise programs to build strength and flexibility. If possible, develop a program that allows you to walk outside safely.

- Physical therapy can help with many conditions, including chronic pain, arthritis, fractures or injuries, balance issues, recovery after surgery, recovery of skills after a stroke or heart attack, wound care, and joint injuries or pain. You should treat physical therapy as a vital part of your fitness program. If you are dealing with a chronic condition or disability, be sure to ask your doctor for a physical therapy referral.

Specific Health Conditions

- Research has demonstrated the beneficial effects of exercise both as a preventive strategy and as a therapeutic treatment for several illnesses, including arthritis, cancer, chronic obstructive pulmonary disease, hypertension, osteoporosis, stroke and heart attack, type II diabetes, and others. In short, across the board, exercise can

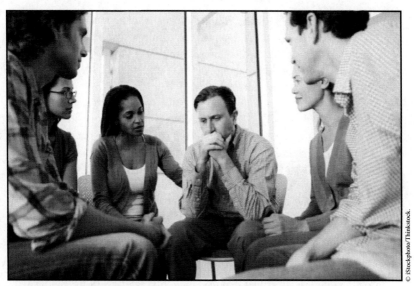

For those dealing with a chronic or acute health condition, a support group offers the opportunity to talk with others who are facing similar challenges.

improve both your health and your quality of life when you are dealing with a chronic condition.

- Research has consistently demonstrated that individuals who regularly exercise experience a lower risk rate for many cancers, including colon and breast cancer. Further, exercise appears to improve quality of life for individuals undergoing cancer treatment and to support life satisfaction and well-being in cancer survivors.
  - Cancer can be particularly challenging because patients have to deal with both the pain of the disorder and the pain of treatment. Exercise can help with both. For instance, many cancer therapies cause fatigue, but research shows that cancer patients who regularly do moderate exercise experience 40% to 50% less fatigue. Exercise also supports mood and helps treat the anxiety and depression that often accompany a cancer diagnosis.

o Exercise for those fighting cancer should be moderate; the body needs to focus on healing, not repairing itself after exhaustive exercise. Moderate exercise can have a major impact on quality of life during cancer treatment, and after treatment, exercise can help prevent recurrence.

- After a stroke or heart attack, rehabilitation serves three goals: (1) to regain the previous level of ability, (2) to prevent another cardiovascular event, and (3) to improve cardiovascular fitness.
  o Multiple controlled studies have shown that exercise after a stroke or heart attack can help individuals regain functional abilities and reduce the risk of future cardiovascular events.

  o Physical therapy to support rebuilding abilities for activities of daily living is important, as is aerobic exercise, in particular, walking. Strength, flexibility, and balance training are all key components of an exercise plan after a stroke or heart attack.

Safety Considerations
- Before beginning an exercise program, discuss your condition with your doctor to address concerns, contraindications, and precautions. Note that a primary-care physician may have minimal training in the use of exercise for symptom management; if necessary, ask for a referral to a qualified physical therapist or exercise physiologist.

- Work with a trained professional who has a solid background in exercise science and experience working with your condition. This professional will help you develop a program that is individualized to your health condition and current fitness level.

- Make sure you have the right equipment to support your health needs. For instance, if you're diabetic, you need to be particularly careful with your feet; get good walking shoes fitted by a podiatrist who works with diabetic patients. Talk with your exercise professional and your doctor about any logistical considerations or special equipment needs.

- Discuss chronic and acute pain with your doctor and exercise professional. If you have a chronic condition, you don't want to push yourself and make your condition worse. However, if you experience chronic pain, it is likely that you will have some discomfort as a result of exercise, at least initially. You will need to learn to distinguish an appropriate level of discomfort from a worrisome level of pain.

- Finally, discuss realistic expectations with your doctor and exercise professional. What can you reasonably expect from an exercise program, based on your condition? Will exercise prevent a decline in functionality? Could exercise potentially lead to an improvement in your symptoms? Exercise may not be able to undo a health condition you're dealing with, but it can always improve the quality of life you have.

Suggested Reading

American College of Sports Medicine, ed., *ACSM's Exercise Management for Persons with Chronic Diseases and Disabilities.*

Gardner-Nix and Kabat-Zinn, *The Mindfulness Solution to Pain.*

National Center on Health, Physical Activity, and Disability, www.ncpad.org.

Activities and Assignments

Reflect on a chronic condition that you are currently dealing with. If you don't have anything, consider yourself lucky and do the reflective exercises hypothetically so that you're prepared for any future issues. First, think about what fears you have and what wants you are clinging to that may be limiting your ability to be active. Write down all the fears and desires that are holding you back.

Think about how you can address your fears positively and move your desires to the category of "hopeful possibilities."

Challenges—Illness and Chronic Pain
Lecture 10—Transcript

How you respond to illness, disability, or a chronic health condition will play a large part in determining your quality of life for the rest of your life. When it is hardest, is when you just might need exercise the most. Your ability to maintain or rebuild your physical independence requires you to be motivated to work through physical activity even when it is difficult. It requires a multifaceted approach of self-care, the right medical support, and social support from friends and family. This is not a time when you can do it alone. However, while you need to accept help from your loved ones in a time of illness, at the end of the day, you have to take responsibility to work through the discomfort so that you can rebuild your health and strength. How you respond can lead to drastically different outcomes.

For example, falls are the leading cause of fatal and nonfatal injuries to adults age 65 and older. Some studies state that as many as 33 percent of those who fracture a hip will die within a year, and as many as 75 percent of those who were independent prior to a hip fracture will neither walk independently nor be living independently a year after the fracture. So if you fall and fracture a hip, complying with physical therapy and getting yourself back up and moving will be key to preventing early death, and reestablishing independence and quality of life.

When you're young, pain usually is an indicator that something is wrong and you need to stop. This is acute pain: pain that comes on suddenly, is sharp in quality, and indicates an injury. Acute pain occurs when you break a bone, strain a muscle, have dental work or surgery, or an illness. Acute pain goes away when the underlying condition has been healed. Once the bone repairs, or you have the root canal, or your surgical wounds heal, acute pain diminishes.

Sometimes, though, pain lingers. The initial injury has healed, but its effects remain in the nervous system. Chronic pain occurs through a variety of conditions; for instance, pain may be the primary symptom of a condition such as arthritis or fibromyalgia, or it may be part of a variety of symptoms in a condition such as Parkinson's. Chronic pain can be a consequence of complications in a condition such as advanced diabetes, where many individuals suffer from chronic foot pain. Injuries or illnesses such as shingles can leave lingering pain. Skin conditions—eczema, psoriasis—can cause chronic discomfort and pain. As we get older, sometimes the body heals more slowly, and the acute pain of surgery can lead to chronic pain in the surgical area: a shoulder or knee or hip that never quite feels right again.

Chronic pain affects more Americans than diabetes, heart disease, and cancer combined. Approximately 1 in 4 adults experiences chronic pain, with the most common types of chronic pain being low back pain (27 percent of people), severe headaches or migraines (15 percent), neck pain (15 percent), and facial ache or pain (4 percent). Chronic pain may affect quality of life and life satisfaction more than any other single factor. Sixty percent of chronic pain sufferers say that chronic pain reduces their enjoyment of life, 77 percent report feelings of depression, and 86 percent report that pain affects their sleep. Fifty-one percent of those with chronic pain feel that they have little or no control over their pain. And if you remember back to Lecture 1, when we discussed locus of control, if you don't feel like you have control over the outcomes in your life, that can have negative impacts on your health and well-being.

The effects of chronic pain can be long lasting. Some research studies indicate that the average individual with chronic pain will suffer for seven years, and that over a fifth of individuals will endure pain for more than 20 years. In the U.S., we spend more than $635 billion per year on chronic pain. Some of that money goes to pain medicine, including strong pain medicines such as opiates. Unfortunately, even opiates reduce chronic pain by, at best, 20 to 30 percent. They also come with risks: Long-term use of opiates can increase your risk of falls, and as we just discussed, falls in particular can be dangerous for older adults and set up a cascade of negative health consequences.

Opiates can also be addictive, and even lead to an increased sensitivity to pain, leading you to need more and more pain medicine to manage your pain. My grandmother had severe pain towards the end of her life, which led to higher and higher dose of opiates just to help her get through the day, and even with them, she still suffered. Even common over-the-counter pain medicines such as non-steroidal anti-inflammatories can lead to other health consequences and side effects, such as wear and tear on the lining of the stomach.

If you break a bone and go to the emergency room, or if you have surgery, your doctor will ask you to rate your pain on a scale of 1 to 10. This is to help them get a sense of the acute pain and make the right decisions about pain medicines to support you during the acute period of injury. The focus with acute pain is on rest and recovery. In contrast, physicians specializing in chronic pain recommend a more holistic approach. Instead of asking about pain levels on a scale of 1 to 10, they will ask you what you want to do, but can't do, because of your pain. The focus is on pain management and improving independence and ability. The treatment approach will focus on education about what pain is, support to improve your social support networks and guidance to help you develop an appropriate program of physical activity and exercise. The focus with chronic pain is helping you live an active life in spite of the pain.

Pain isn't just pain. It's a multidimensional experience, with four key aspects. The physiological-sensory dimension is your body's internal response to pain. The affect dimension is your emotional response to pain. The cognitive dimension is your attitudes and beliefs about pain. The behavioral dimension is the actions you take when pain occurs. So when you physically experience pain, you experience it within the context of your beliefs about pain, and your emotional response to pain, and those help determine how you react to that pain. However, just because a component of pain is in your head, that doesn't make it any less real. Chronic pain is difficult and can be debilitating, so you need the right support to work through so that you can live an active life.

Research indicates that a multi-dimensional approach to pain management is the most effect strategy for helping reduce pain and improve function. For instance, when individuals with chronic pain receive education about pain, including its components and psychological strategies for coping with pain, they experience improved attitudes and self-efficacy, and actually experience reduced pain. Research has found that education programs that focus on understanding and coping strategies may actually be as effective as non-steroidal anti-inflammatories in reducing pain, without the potential side effects of pain medicine. Social support, and education of family members or caregivers, can also be an important part of the pain-management process.

Physical activity may actually be one of the most effective treatments for managing chronic pain. Exercise can reduce the experience of pain and improve functional independence. To make the contrast clear if you have the acute pain of an injury, you need to rest and let the injury heal. If you are dealing with chronic pain, you need to be active to help yourself work through that chronic pain. To improve the potential for positive outcomes in pain management via exercise, it's important for you to have flexible goals that you can adapt based on your pain level or changes in the state of your condition. You also need to pace yourself, and be part of the decision-making process about your exercise program, and then work with a trained professional who has experience working with chronic pain in general and your condition in particular.

Chronic pain is often accompanied by chronic fatigue; remember, 86 percent of people with chronic pain don't sleep well. So if you have chronic pain, you may feel like you're too tired to exercise. This can also occur in conditions, such as multiple sclerosis or chronic fatigue syndrome, where fatigue is a primary symptom of the chronic condition. However, research does show that gentle forms of exercise, for instance, mindfulness fitness practices like yoga, or water aerobics and gentle swimming, can actually improve energy and vigor, and reduce pain and fatigue, in individuals with chronic pain and chronic fatigue. In fact, inactivity may actually exacerbate the symptoms of chronic pain and chronic fatigue, and lead to a worsening of the condition.

Mindfulness activities can be helpful in particular with chronic pain management. First, mindfulness fitness practices like yoga and Tai Chi are very gentle, so you can participate with low risk of injury. They also help you find awareness of the present moment, so that you can learn how to better manage fear or anxiety. Often with chronic pain, the current moment of pain is tolerable, but our fear is that it will never end, and that fear becomes unbearable. Mindfulness strategies help you come back to the present moment, so that you can break out of the fear cycle. If you are dealing with chronic pain, I encourage you to revisit Lecture 6 on mindfulness practices, and also try the yoga, Qigong, and relaxation active lectures. The five-minute Reiki practice session specifically focuses on using the power of deliberate touch to calm your fears and bring you back to the present moment.

The power of touch can be quite powerful in helping you cope with chronic pain. Several research studies have found that complementary therapies such as massage and acupuncture can be helpful in coping with chronic pain. Connection to others and physical touch are both very helpful. Oxytocin is a hormone, which has sometimes been called the love or bonding hormone. Oxytocin is released during childbirth, during breastfeeding, and during orgasm, and it plays a role in bonding and the formation of trust and love. Physical contact also releases oxytocin. Preliminary research has found that oxytocin may be helpful for reducing pain: In one study, oxytocin put into the nose reduced headache pain. Gentle connective touch can be helpful in reducing pain because the body produces oxytocin in response to that touch.

I have my own issues of chronic pain, from a variety of chronic conditions. I'm faithful to self-care, but sometimes, even with good, consistent self-care, the pain wins. Sometimes fatigue or stress can throw all of my self-care efforts out the window, and I wake up the next morning and I can't turn my head. Then it takes weeks of the same diligent self-care before the pain goes away again.

If you have chronic pain, use exercise to help you manage it, but don't beat yourself up when it doesn't always work. There are some schools of thought that say we create our health and everything is in our head. Throw that out the window; you don't need the guilt. When the pain flares, you could focus your energy on beating yourself up and wondering what you did wrong to create it, or you can focus your energy on how you're going to work through it and get back into control. Focus on the positive outcome you want, not the negative outcome you're trying to avoid or overcome. Like our healthy role-model centenarians, we are doing our best to stay positive and focus on what we can actually change.

There's a lot you can do to stay active, regardless of your health condition. Let's talk through some strategies you can use for various levels of mobility. For instance, if you are in the hospital or restricted to bed, you can still move to keep up your strength and keep yourself active. Moving when and how you can will keep you from putting too much pressure on any one spot of the body, so that you can help prevent skin ulcers and bedsores. While you're on bed rest, be realistic and be safe—cooperate with your doctors to plan the best recovery possible. Work to stay active and engaged, and collaborate with the physical therapists and occupational therapists who want to help you get back on your feet as soon as possible. Remember to be your own advocate; you may have to ask for support and referrals. In some cases your doctor may be used to working with people who don't want to push themselves, so be aware of that, and ask for what you need to get healthy again so that you get the support you need.

If you're in bed, on bed rest or in the hospital, here are some strategies you can still do to stay active. For instance, in bed you can use hand-gripper balls, move your hands, keeping up your hand strength. Sit up whenever you can, even if it's sitting up in bed, lifting the bed up, being upright is still more work than lying flat and it gives your body a different position than when you're flat on your back to sleep. Do as much as you can for yourself: brushing your teeth uses your upper arms; feeding yourself so you're still working your arms, your forearms; putting on your own shirt and socks; lifting your arms over your head to get a shirt on; reaching down to your foot to get your socks on. These are small movements that keep your blood flowing and your muscles engaged.

You can also do gentle stretches of your neck, arms, and shoulders. For instance, you can look to your left and hold the stretch, 5, 6 nice deep breaths, opening up the side of the neck. Take the other side. Do these right now while we're talking. Look to your right, breathing here, nice long stretch, and come back to center. You can take the ear to the shoulder, opening up the other parts of the neck, taking the right ear to the shoulder, long stretch. And the other side. They're simple things, but they're great things to do when you're in bed to just keep some movement, some bloodflow. You can stretch your arms up, lifting up towards the ceiling and then stretching towards the left, stretching towards the right. Nice long stretch, and then you can try stretching left, and you're lengthening up through the side; and you could stretch right, lengthening the side, nice and open. And you can roll your shoulders back, and then shrug up and down. Again these are simple things, but they keep you moving.

When you're in bed if it's safe for you to move your legs, every hour that you're awake, spend a few minutes lifting a leg, pointing, flexing your toes to move the blood flow in the lower parts of your legs. Lift one leg up off the bed, hold the lift, and then relax, lift the other leg. It'll keep your lower body moving, prevent clots, prevent edema in the legs, just to keep things moving in your body. Deliberate breathing can help you maintain lung capacity and keep your lungs from getting weak or getting fluid in them. Your medical staff may actually have you breathe into a device throughout the day so that they ensure your lungs are clear, particularly if you've recently had surgery. You can also do simple, abdominal breathing as a simple exercise to keep your lungs strong.

We've done this before in the course, but let's take a minute to reiterate, focus on our breathing. Put your hands on your stomach, take a nice deep inhalation, breathing into the lower lobes of your lungs, let your stomach relax into your hands as you inhale. And then as you exhale, belly button back towards the spine, pushing the air out of your body through the nose, in and out through the nose, always, but breathing gently into the lungs, breathing with your body into your abdomen, deep breaths, one more, inhale. Exhale. Simple and gentle but something you can do if you're in bed to keep engaging the core muscles of your body and making sure that you're really using your lungs to keep your breathing strong.

If you're able to sit up in a chair or a wheelchair, you can do all of the exercises we just discussed, and add some additional strategies. You can work on your strength by using hand weights, resistance bands, or even water bottles or soup cans, to do upper-body strengthening exercises. If you have some use of your legs, you can do exercises in the chair, such as leg lifts or stretches with resistance bands. The fitness fundamentals, chair yoga, and Qigong active lectures all provide examples of exercises you can do while seated.

You also still need to do endurance exercise, if possible. Some physical therapy facilities offer arm bicycling or rowing machines, which you may be able to use. If you have access to an adapted swimming pool that can help you in, this is a great option for exercise. If you have built up upper-body strength, you can use a manual wheelchair powered by your arms: Traveling a distance by arm power can provide a cardiovascular workout through repetitive, large muscle activity. If you are able to walk with the use of a walker, it's important for you to stay as active as you can to either maintain the walking capacity you have, or, if possible, rebuild your strength for independent walking. You can do both the bed-based activities and chair-based exercise programs to support you in building strength and flexibility, and then also spend some time each day and deliberately focusing on getting up, standing up from a chair and sitting down in a chair. Remember we talked about standing up and sitting down without using your arms. Even if you're using your arms, work on getting up, getting down, so you're building, strengthening your legs, developing improved abilities in your thighs and your glutes. Hold the chair for balance and support, but concentrate on gradually reducing how much weight your arms hold, and moving more and more of that to your legs.

Also be deliberate about a walking program to build endurance of your lungs and legs. Use your walker or your cane for your safety and balance. If you feel embarrassed that you need a cane or a walker, let go of that emotion and accept the help you need. You are better off to use a cane or walker for balance and keep moving independently, than to skip the walker, lose your balance, fall, and end up in a hospital bed. You can maintain your independence and health with a walker or a cane, but it's much harder to maintain your independence in a hospital bed.

I've talked a couple of times about my grandma, and when her balance and hips got worse, she needed a walker, but she still went for a two-mile walk every day with our family with a walker. It was a slower walk, but it kept her up and moving, and she got fresh air and sunshine. We went for daily walks with her until her last six weeks of life—she kept walking up until that point. As part of my master's thesis research, I offered different exercise interventions at a senior living community. For one group, we went for walks three days per week. We walked in a group, I walked with them to ensure that each participant had the safety and support they needed. We walked on a paved trail around the facility so that there were no potential risk hazards.

Some individuals walked independently, some people needed canes, and some people needed walkers, but everyone increased their walking speed and strength over the course of the activity.

Work as hard as you can, for as long as you can, to keep walking. So what if you use a cane or a walker, so what if you get slow; you're still walking, moving, you're active. Try to avoid the siren call of the electric wheelchair if you can. In my experience with older adults, very rarely have I seen someone move from a walker to an electric chair and then back to the walker. Every time I see someone make the decision to get the electric wheelchair because their doctor has talked them into it, told them they are entitled to it and insurance will pay for it, I worry, because it can become a downward spiral from there. Try to keep walking if you can.

Physical therapy and occupational therapy are vital. They can be so important in helping you rebuild basic skills and skills for daily living after an injury, surgery, or illness. Physical therapy can help with many conditions, including chronic pain, arthritis, fractures, injuries, balance issues, recovery after surgery, regaining skills after a stroke or heart attack, wound care, and joint injuries or pain. It is an important part of recovery, and you should treat it as a vital part of your fitness program. If you are dealing with a chronic condition or disability, and your doctor does not offer, be sure to ask him or her for a physical therapy referral.

Adapted and modified physical fitness programs can help you recover more quickly, and retain greater independence, during illness, chronic health conditions, and in spite of disabilities. Modified fitness programs are key to keep you active and either maintain or rebuild your independence. Research has demonstrated the beneficial effects of exercise both as a preventative strategy and as a therapeutic treatment for several illnesses, including arthritis, cancer, chronic obstructive pulmonary disease, chronic renal failure, cognitive impairment, congestive heart failure, coronary artery disease, depression, disability, hypertension, osteoporosis, peripheral vascular disease, stroke and heart attack, and type-2 diabetes. In short, across the board, exercise can both improve your health and help improve your quality of life when you are dealing with a chronic condition.

Let's talk about cancer for a moment. Exercise has multiple impacts on cancer. Research has consistently demonstrated that individuals who regularly exercise experience a lower risk rate for many cancers, including colon and breast cancer. As well, exercise appears to improve quality of life for individuals undergoing cancer treatment, and it supports life satisfaction and well-being in cancer survivors. Cancer can be particularly challenging because you have to deal with both the agony of the disorder and the agony of treatment. Exercise can help with both. For instance, many cancer therapies cause fatigue, but research shows that cancer patients who regularly do moderate exercise experience 40–50 percent less fatigue. Exercise also supports mood and helps treat the anxiety and depression that often accompany a cancer diagnosis.

When fighting cancer, exercise should be moderate; this isn't the time to train for a marathon, because you need your body to focus on healing, not repairing itself after exhaustive exercise. However, moderate exercise can have a major impact on your quality of life during cancer treatment. After treatment, exercise can help prevent recurrence; some studies have shown that gaining weight after cancer treatment can increase the likelihood of a recurrence, particularly for breast, colon, and prostate cancer, and that exercise that prevents weight gain can help reduce the likelihood of recurrence. It can also help manage the ongoing psychological stress of wondering if the cancer will stay in remission.

In the U.S., more than 795,000 people have a stroke each year. Another 715,000 Americans will have a heart attack. More than half of those who have a stroke will die within eight years, often from another cardiovascular illness; a third of strokes and heart attacks are a recurrent event. After a stroke or heart attack, rehabilitation serves three goals: to regain the previous level of ability, to prevent another cardiovascular event, and to improve cardiovascular fitness. Exercise helps with all three of these goals, and multiple controlled studies have shown that exercise after a stroke or heart attack can help individuals regain functional abilities and reduce the risk for future cardiovascular events. Physical therapy to support rebuilding abilities for activities of daily living is important. Also key is aerobic activity; in particular, walking. Individuals who need support while walking can walk on a treadmill, using the rails, to support balance and reduce risk of falling.

Strength training, flexibility, and balance training are all key components of an exercise plan after a stroke or heart attack.

If you are dealing with a chronic or acute health condition, social support is an important part of your recovery. Unfortunately, your friends and family may not really understand what you are going through, and when they want to help, they may not know how. Consider joining a support group so that you can talk with people who are going through the same condition, and who truly understand what you are experiencing. If you are dealing with a chronic condition, close family members may want to join a caretaker support group, so that they have a better sense of support and a clearer understanding for what you both are experiencing. When your friends and family want to help, be helpful to them by letting them know what you need. Explain what kind of support you would like, and what you don't want. Give them specific guidance and feedback about how to be there for you in the best way.

You may have some friends and family members who can't talk about your health condition, or who disappoint or disappear. Some people are afraid of illness, almost as if they have an unconscious fear that pain or disability are contagious. This isn't your fault. They have their own reasons and their own issues why they can't handle your pain and discomfort, so focus on your own healing, and on the people who want to be there to support you. If you are dealing with a chronic or acute condition, you may find that exercise is an effective treatment modality, either as primary therapy or as a supportive adjunct to therapy. But you need to follow some safety guidelines: Discuss your condition with your doctor, and address any concerns, contraindications, or precautions with regard to exercise. Do know that a primary care physician may have very minimal training in the use of exercise for symptom management, so ask for a referral to a qualified physical therapist or exercise physiologist for additional support. Some hospital systems now have wellness programs in place, and may offer either individual or group sessions with trained exercise professionals focused on the management of specific conditions.

Make sure you work with a trained professional, who has a solid background in exercise science, and experience and training working with your condition. Your program should be individualized to your health condition and your current fitness level. There is never a one-size-fits-all program in exercise, but when you are using exercise as an adjunct to medical care, it is even more important that your exercise program truly fits you. The type, duration, intensity, and frequency of exercise should all fit your life and your comfort level. Also, your environment, resources, and social support network should be taken into account. If you can't drive, you need to consider transportation as a factor—you can't take an exercise class at a facility if you can't get there. Develop a plan that supports you in adhering to it, because you will only experience a program's benefits if you can actually participate.

Have the right equipment to support your health needs. If you're diabetic, you need to be particularly careful with your feet, so get good, solid, safe walking shoes, fitted by a podiatrist who works with diabetic patients. If you're going through chemotherapy for cancer, your immune system isn't as strong, so avoid communal hot tubs at the gym, avoid crowded exercise classes where you might be exposed to other people with colds or other viruses. If you have a heart condition, yoga is great, but make sure it's a gentle yoga class, and avoid a heated yoga class, which is not safe for anyone with hypertension or other heart concerns. Talk with your exercise professional and your doctor about any logistical considerations or equipment needs.

Discuss chronic and acute pain with your doctor and your exercise professional. If you have a chronic condition, you don't want to push yourself and make your condition worse. However, if you experience chronic pain, it is likely that there will be some discomfort due to exercise, at least initially. Research indicates that regular exercise can improve your experience of pain, so that overtime you will experience less pain. You will need to learn to distinguish an appropriate level of discomfort from a worrisome level of pain. You can also learn coping strategies such as breathing and distraction techniques to help you work through initial discomfort. You also want to discuss realistic expectations with your doctor and your exercise professional. What can you reasonably expect, based on your condition? Will exercise prevent a decline in functionality? Could it potentially lead to an improvement in your symptoms? For some conditions, for instance, amyotrophic lateral sclerosis or ALS, it is unlikely that exercise will prevent the condition from progressing. However, physical therapy and appropriate exercise can help an individual with ALS maintain as much functionality and quality of life as possible.

A few years ago, I received an email from a nice gentleman named Bob. He had ALS, and a friend had given him my chair yoga DVD as a gift. We had a really nice email correspondence back and forth, and he shared that he couldn't do all the exercises, but overall it helped him feel calm and he really liked the breathing exercises. Months, months later his friend wrote to share that Bob had passed, but that he'd done the yoga DVD every day until the end.

So it's important to have a sense of what's possible for you. Exercise may not be able to undo a health condition you're dealing with. But it can always improve the quality of life that you have. Maybe you didn't expect to have this health condition; it doesn't feel fair. Don't let your expectations of what life should have been get in the way of you making the most of what is. Don't let yourself get stuck in mourning what you've lost and what you used to have. Try to move forward with a sense of optimism about what you can still have. The right exercise program can help you make the most of what is.

For today's takeaway, reflect on a chronic condition which you are currently dealing with. If you don't have anything, consider yourself lucky. Do a hypothetical exercise so you're prepared for anything in the future. First, think about what fears you have, what wants you are clinging to, what may be limiting your ability to be active. Are you afraid of falling or worried about pain? Are you angry that you can't do something you used to do? Write down all the fears and "wants" that are holding you back.

Next, think about how you can address those fears positively, and move "wants" to "hopeful possibilities." If you're afraid of falling, what steps could you take to address that, so that you can exercise in a safe way? If you're worried about discomfort, what can you do to have a lower likelihood of pain? For the "wants,": Maybe you used to love hiking. Can you start with gentle walks on level ground? Or start with walking in a pool, to rebuild range of motion? Can you do other things out in nature to get fresh air and sunshine? Focus on making the most of what is, instead of mourning what you've lost.

If you suffer from a chronic condition, it may sometimes feel like life isn't fair. As my grandmother's pain got worse, sometimes she would ask rhetorically, "Why am I made to suffer?" Life isn't fair. It's hard not to feel like you're being punished by your suffering. There are no Pollyanna magic cures: Exercise isn't going to make it all go away and get better. It's not going to erase your pain. But it will give you skills and strategies to improve your quality of life, and help you make the most of what you do have. So let go of what you've lost, focus on all that you have, and look towards the possibilities that are still in front of you.

Small Steps—A Path to Big Benefits
Lecture 11

A s you start to add more physical activity into your life, you will begin to notice its benefits. You may be a little less tired in the morning and find it's easier to get out of bed. You may also notice that you are less irritable throughout the day. Your waistband may be a little looser or your briefcase may seem a little lighter. These small benefits add up and combine with other, more subtle improvements, of which you might not even be aware. In this lecture, we'll discuss the benefits of physical activity to provide you with one more source of motivation to keep moving.

Health Components for Long Life

- As we discussed in Lecture 1, there is no fountain of youth that will keep you from aging, but health-promoting decisions, such as incorporating regular physical activity into your life, will have a profound impact on the way you age and the degree of health and independence you maintain throughout your lifespan.

- According to research, the physiological factors most often associated with longevity and successful aging are low blood pressure; low BMI; low levels of fat around the waistline; preserved glucose tolerance; and a protective blood lipid profile, with low triglycerides, low LDL cholesterol, and high HDL cholesterol. The one activity that consistently helps to promote all these health characteristics is exercise.

- Based on all the positive health benefits of physical activity and exercise, the ACSM indicates that physical activity is a lifestyle factor that "discriminates between individuals who have and have not experienced successful aging." In fact, cardiovascular fitness levels may actually predict your likelihood of becoming functionally dependent.

Physical Benefits of Activity

- If you have already begun to incorporate more physical activity into your life, one benefit you have likely already experienced is improved energy and stamina. It seems counterintuitive when you think you're too tired to exercise, but exercise actually increases energy and vigor and reduces fatigue.

- Exercise also supports weight management and reduces the risk of obesity. In particular, it reduces both overall weight and the fat mass that is more dangerous, such as the internal fat mass around the abdomen. It's also true that a leaner, fitter body burns more calories even when not exercising. For instance, some studies have found that 12 to 26 weeks of resistance training can increase metabolic rate by as much as 9%.

- Exercise improves your hormonal profile, decreasing levels of resting cortisol, a hormone that can increase as a result of stress and can be related to weight gain.

- Not only can exercise reduce blood pressure and cholesterol levels, but it also reduces overall risk for cardiovascular disease. People who exercise regularly are at a lower risk for stroke and heart attack. Even without dietary changes, exercise improves the body's ability to clear lipids and, in particular, triglycerides from circulation after a meal and to use fat as fuel during moderate-intensity exercise.

- The same is true for diabetes; regular exercise reduces the risk of developing type II diabetes and reduces the risk of serious complications for those who are diabetics. Benefits for diabetics, such as improved glycemic control and insulin action, occur even without dietary changes. Of course, when exercise and appropriate dietary changes are combined, outcomes improve dramatically.

- Exercise reduces the risk of osteoporosis and the risk of fractures. Low-intensity weight-bearing activities, such as walking, can have a modest effect on bone density at the hip and spine in postmenopausal women. Weight-bearing activities also counteract age-related bone loss (0.5%–1% in sedentary postmenopausal women) that otherwise occurs. Higher-intensity weight-bearing activities, such as climbing stairs or brisk walking (practiced for at least 1 to 2 years), can have stronger impacts on bone density.

- Of course, exercise also helps increase strength. Regular resistance training can improve muscular strength at least 25% and as much as 100% or more, actually doubling your strength.
  - o Muscle strength is the amount of force you can generate, while muscle power is the ability to generate as much force as possible as fast as possible. Aging often reduces muscular power even more than muscular strength. Fortunately, research has found that resistance training can lead to substantial increases in muscular power in older adults.

  - o Muscular endurance, which is the capacity to use muscular strength repeatedly over time, is also important in maintaining functional independence as we get older. Muscular endurance affects your ability to walk independently, carry your own groceries, and so on. Your level of muscular endurance may determine your travel range in older adulthood.

- Individuals who exercise regularly are more able to cope with back pain, headaches, and other chronic pain conditions. As we discussed in the last lecture, exercise also offers many therapeutic benefits for treatment and management of health conditions, including coronary heart disease, hypertension, type II diabetes, elevated cholesterol, osteoporosis, osteoarthritis, and so on.

Psychological Benefits of Activity
- As we've seen, both improved physical fitness and regular participation in physical activity are associated with improved psychological health. For instance, exercise supports improved cognitive function. A single bout of exercise can improve cognitive performance; promote clearer thinking; and create immediate improvements in memory, reaction time, and attention.

- With regular exercise, you can improve your memory and perception and reduce the risk of cognitive impairment and dementia with aging. Exercise can even slow the onset of dementia; in contrast, becoming physically inactive can increase the risk and onset of cognitive decline.

- Over the last century, mortality rates have decreased and life expectancy has increased, but some researchers have questioned whether those later years provide quality of life. According to the Centers for Disease Control and Prevention, after age 65, the risk of developing Alzheimer's doubles every 5 years. By age 85, between 25% and 50% of individuals will exhibit signs of Alzheimer's. Even though dementia is common in older adults, it is not a normal part of the aging process. Healthy lifestyle choices and exercise can improve your chances of preventing dementia into older age.

- In fact, your fitness level can actually help predict your risk of cognitive decline. Your walking speed and whether or not you can walk 1 kilometer—about 0.6 miles—are associated with cognitive impairment. There are also associations between cognitive impairment and other routine physical measures, such as grip strength and whether or not you can stand up out of a chair.

- Aerobic exercise is key for psychological health, but even better outcomes occur when you combine aerobic exercise, resistance training, and flexibility training with mental exercise programs. The greatest effects on cognition seem to occur when exercise sessions exceed 30 minutes. Exercise seems to influence executive control in particular, such as planning, scheduling, working memory, and task coordination.

- Exercise is also associated with improved work efficiency, reduced absenteeism from work, and reduced work errors. Not only will you perform better at work if you exercise, but you might even earn more. One study found that exercising 3 times per week is correlated with a 6% to 10% increase in wages. In contrast, another study found that obese women earned 18% less than women of normal

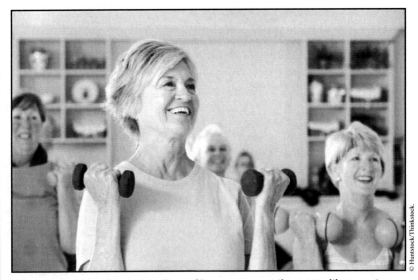

Research has found that regardless of how many negative or positive events you experience in a day, even a single session of exercise will improve your mood.

© Hunstock/Thinkstock.

weight, and a third study found that overweight women have a total family income of 25% less than women of normal weight.

- Regular exercise helps to reduce stress, anxiety, anger, and depression and reduces the risk of developing clinical anxiety and depression. In fact, exercise can reduce symptoms of clinical depression in older adults by as much as 88%. Adults who are inactive are more likely to be depressed.

- Overall, the National Institute of Mental Health has concluded that physical fitness is positively associated with mental health and well-being, that exercise specifically helps reduce stress and anxiety, that exercise helps reduce mild to moderate depression, and that even in severe cases of clinical anxiety and depression, exercise is a useful adjunct to psychotherapy and other forms of clinical treatment.

- Nine weeks of regular exercise seems to be the point at which patients experience significant outcomes in reducing depression.

In fact, a longer-term exercise program can be as effective as psychotherapy or medication in treating depression. Long-term studies have shown that reductions in anxiety are not connected to physical changes in fitness levels. Even if you don't feel as if you're increasing your fitness or losing weight, exercise still has a positive impact on your mood.

- Other psychological benefits of regular exercise include improvement in life satisfaction, overall well-being, and quality of life; increased positive affect; improved body image; higher self-esteem; and a greater sense of self-efficacy, that is, your belief in your ability to accomplish specific tasks.

Promoting Psychological Health

- Research has identified several key components of exercise programs that promote psychological health. First, the exercise program needs to include rhythmic abdominal breathing. Aerobic exercise, such as swimming or walking, can do this, but so can mindful fitness practices, such as yoga and Tai Chi.

- Second, the exercise program must provide a relative absence of interpersonal competition. Although competition may be fun and exciting for some people, it can also lead to overtraining, pressure to win, and a sense of social evaluation. Research shows that noncompetitive forms of exercise are most likely to promote psychological health.

- Exercise that is done in a closed and predictable environment is most likely to promote psychological health. This type of environment varies depending on your experience and expectations; it may be a pool for someone who is comfortable swimming, or it may be a golf course for someone who regularly plays golf. Generally speaking, self-paced environments in which you have a good understanding of what to expect allow you to focus on the activity you're performing without distraction.

- Fourth, to experience consistent improvement in well-being, you need to exercise for at least 20 minutes a day, at least 2 to 3 times per week. Note that the amount of exercise you need to promote mental health is less than what you need for physical health.

- Finally, the most critical component of an exercise program intended to promote psychological health may be the most obvious thing you're unlikely to think of: You need to enjoy it. We often associate exercise with something we need to put on our to-do list and slog through. If you find an exercise program you truly enjoy, you're more likely both to do it and to benefit from it.

Suggested Reading

Chodzko-Zajko, et al., "American College of Sports Medicine, Position Stand: Exercise and Physical Activity for Older Adults."

U.S. Department of Health and Human Services, "2008 Physical Activity Guidelines for Americans."

Activities and Assignments

What are the health characteristics you want to promote through exercise? Identify the personal health needs that will most inspire you to keep going. Focus on framing your motivators in a positive context rather than a negative one.

Reflect on your experience with this course so far. What benefits have you already experienced from exercise?

Assess your own level of competitiveness. When, where, and how do you compete against others? What's the internal motivation for that feeling of competition? How does competition affect your fitness? What can you do to better support yourself in giving up that inner urge for competition so that you can be more open to trying new things and enjoying them just for the sake of enjoyment?

Small Steps—A Path to Big Benefits
Lecture 11—Transcript

We've had quite a journey. I hope that, by now, you've tried some of the active sessions, and that you have put your improved understanding of fitness and fitness principles to work. If so, you are likely feeling some benefits. Perhaps you are a little less tired in the morning, and it's a little easier to get out of bed. Maybe you don't need quite as many cups of coffee to get through the day. Perhaps you've noticed that you are less irritable, less likely to get frustrated with your spouse or angry at work. Maybe your waistband's a little looser, maybe your briefcase seem a little lighter. Maybe you can reach the high shelves in the grocery store a little easier. Those small benefits add up, and there have also been other, more subtle improvements, of which you might not even be aware. In this lecture, we'll discuss the benefits of physical activity to provide you with one more source of motivation to keep moving.

To put what we have been doing into context, here is a statement from the American College of Sports Medicine Position Stand on Exercise and Physical Activity for Older Adults: "Although no amount of physical activity can stop the biological aging process, there is evidence that regular exercise can minimize the physiological effects of an otherwise sedentary lifestyle and increase active life expectancy by limiting the development and progression of chronic disease and disabling conditions." So, as we discussed in Lecture 1, there is no fountain of youth that will keep you from aging, but health-promoting decisions like regular physical activity will have a profound impact on the way you age, and how much health and independence you maintain throughout your lifespan.

Let's go back to our centenarians: adults over age 100. They can tell us a lot about the physical health components required to sustain a long healthy life. According to research, the physiological factors most often associated with longevity and successful aging are low blood pressure, low body mass index, low levels of fat around the waistline, preserved glucose tolerance, and a protective blood lipid profile, with low triglycerides and low LDL cholesterol, and high HDL cholesterol. To monitor these aspects of your health, you will need a good relationship with your medical practitioner.

Work with your doctor to determine what your current health risk factors are for each of these indicators, and to determine how often you should test each component.

They sound abstract and complicated, and I don't want you to get obsessed with tracking a few numbers on a lab report. The point, though, is that there is one activity that consistently helps to promote all of those health characteristics that our centenarians share: Exercise. Regular physical activity. Regular physical activity can reduce your blood pressure, it reduces your body mass, it reduces your waistline, it improves your glucose tolerance, which helps prevent or control diabetes, and it improves your cholesterol and triglyceride levels. Based on all of the positive health benefits of physical activity and exercise, the American College of Sports Medicine indicates that physical activity is a lifestyle factor that "discriminates between individuals who have and have not experienced successful aging." In fact, cardiovascular fitness levels may actually predict your likelihood of becoming functionally dependent.

Let's start with the physical benefits of physical activity, and the way exercise can reduce your risk for many diseases. One benefit that you've likely already experienced is improved energy and stamina. It seems counterintuitive when you think you're too tired to exercise, but exercise actually increases energy and vigor, and reduces fatigue. Exercise also supports weight management and reduces the risk of obesity. If you've starting moving, then you have probably noticed that even if the needle on the scale hasn't moved with you, your waistband is a little looser. It doesn't matter what form of exercise you are doing. Aerobic exercise and resistance training both support improved body composition and reduce the risk of obesity.

In fact, exercise reduces both overall weight and the fat mass that is more dangerous, such as the internal fat mass around the abdomen. The benefits on your weight may have less to do with the time you spend exercising and more to do with the way a leaner, fitter body burns calories throughout the rest of the day. For instance, some studies have found that 12–26 weeks of resistance training can increase metabolic rate by as much as 9 percent. Resistance training may also improve your ability to use fat as fuel, which makes it easier for your body to burn off fat stores. Exercise also improves your hormonal profile. Exercise can decrease levels of resting cortisol. We've talked about cortisol before, a hormone which increases due to stress, and elevated cortisol can be related to weight gain.

Exercise also reduces your risk of minor illnesses like colds and flus. Now, as we noted in Lecture 9, when people over train, there is a risk it will compromise their immune system. The most substantial benefits to your immune system are with regular, moderate exercise. We talked also in Lecture 8 about the importance of social networks, how our friends and family can influence our health. One interesting research study found that exercise combined with a good social support network resulted in the lowest level of illness.

Exercise not only reduces your blood pressure and your cholesterol levels, it reduces your overall risk for cardiovascular disease. People who exercise regularly are at a lower risk for stroke and heart attack. Even without dietary changes, exercise improves the body's ability to clear lipids and in particular triglycerides from your circulation after a meal, and to use fat as fuel during moderate intensity exercise. The same is true for diabetics: Regular exercise reduces the risk of developing type-2 diabetes, and reduces the risk of serious complications for those who are diabetics. Benefits for diabetics, like improved glycemic control and insulin action, occur even without dietary changes. Of course, when exercise and appropriate dietary changes are combined, it improves the outcomes drastically. As well, regular exercise can reduce your risk for many cancers, including colon cancer and breast cancer.

Exercise reduces your risk of osteoporosis, and also reduces your risk for fractures. Large-scale studies indicate physical activity in general, and walking in particular, can reduce the risk of osteoporosis-related fractures by 50 percent. Low-intensity weight-bearing activities like walking can have a modest effect on bone density at the hip and spine in postmenopausal women. Low-intensity weight-bearing exercise needs to occur at minimum three to five days per week, for at least a year to have an impact on bone density.

Weight-bearing activities also counteract the age-related losses that would otherwise occur. Normal bone loss is 0.5–1 percent of bone per year in sedentary postmenopausal women. Higher-intensity weight bearing activities, like climbing stairs or brisk walking, for at least one to two years, can have an even stronger impact on bone density. The exercise has to be weight bearing to benefit your bones. So swimming and biking are great exercise for other health conditions; they won't help your bones stay strong. Walking is a fabulous exercise to keep your bones strong. The effects of exercise on bone mass have been documented for men as well. One study found that middle-aged and older men who ran at least nine times per month had lower levels of bone loss in the spine.

The best exercise programs for improving balance and reducing risk of falls combine strength, balance, and flexibility. Tai Chi, Qigong, and yoga are all great options. I encourage you to try the active sessions. For optimal benefits, combine regular practices with walking several times per week. Exercise also helps increase strength. Regular resistance training can improve muscular strength at least 25 percent and as much as more than 100 percent, which means you actually double your strength through regular resistance training.

Muscle strength is the amount of force you can generate, while muscle power is the ability to generate as much force as possible as fast as possible, so muscle power is the speed of your strength. Aging often reduces muscular power even more than muscular strength. Fortunately, research has found that resistance training can lead to substantial increases in muscular power in older adults. Muscular endurance, your capacity to use muscular strength repeatedly over time, is very important in maintaining functional independence, as we get older. Muscular endurance affects your ability to walk independently, to carry your own groceries. In fact, your level of muscular endurance may actually determine your travel range in older adulthood. For instance, will you be confined to your home or a care facility? Or will you still be able to walk steps, and move around without assistance? This can be profound for someone with a health condition that could otherwise limit his or her mobility and freedom.

I had a dear friend named Owen who had epilepsy in his older years. After his wife passed, he was not able to drive by himself. But he was intent and focused on staying independent, so he continued to push himself to walk; he walked several miles each day, which allowed him to continue independently to go to church, to go to the grocery store, and run other errands by himself. He protected his travel range by continuing to move. In fact, he lived independently until his last few years, in his late 80s, when he moved near a niece to live in a care facility. Even if you've started losing some of your muscular endurance, you can get it back. Research has demonstrated that resistance training can increase muscular endurance by as much as 200 percent.

We talked in our last lecture about chronic pain, and the ways that exercise can help both with the conditions that cause chronic pain, and with the management and perception of chronic pain. Individuals who exercise regularly are more able to cope with back pain, headaches, and other chronic pain conditions. As we discussed in our last lecture, exercise offers other therapeutic benefits: supportive treatment and management of conditions, like coronary heart disease, hypertension, peripheral vascular disease, type-2 diabetes, elevated cholesterol, osteoporosis, osteoarthritis, chronic obstructive pulmonary disease, congestive heart failure, constipation, and gastrointestinal disease. All of them can be benefitted and improved by regular exercise.

Let's also talk about the psychological benefits of physical activity. As a society, we don't talk about mental health care as much as we talk about the care of our bodies. But even if we're not talking about, it's affecting us. Mental health problems account for 30 percent of the total days of hospitalization in the U.S., and about 10 percent of medical costs. Individuals with depressions spend 1.5 times more on health care than non-depressed individuals.

The positive thing is that we can promote our own mental health. Both improved physical fitness and regular participation in physical activity are associated with improved psychological health. For instance, exercise supports improved cognitive function. A single bout of exercise can actually improve cognitive performance, promoting clearer thinking, and create immediate improvements in memory, reaction time, and attention. With regular exercise, we can improve our memory, improve our perception, and even reduce our risk of cognitive impairment and dementia with aging. Exercise can slow the onset of dementia; in contrast, becoming physically inactive can increase the risk and onset of cognitive decline.

Over the last century, mortality rates have decreased and life expectancy has increased. Some researchers have questioned whether those later years, those longer years that we're living, are providing quality of life. According to the Centers for Disease Control and Prevention, after age 65, the risk of developing Alzheimer's doubles every five years. By age 85, between 25 and 50 percent of individuals will exhibit signs of Alzheimer's. Even though dementia is common in older adults, it is not a normal part of the aging process. Healthy lifestyle choices and exercise can improve your chances of preventing dementia into older age.In fact, your fitness level can actually help predict your risk of cognitive decline. Your ability to walk can indicate potential cognitive impairment. Researchers have discovered that walking speed and whether or not you can walk 1 kilometer, about 0.6 miles, are associated with cognitive impairment. There are also associations between cognitive impairment and other routine physical measures such as grip strength and whether or not you can stand up out of a chair.

The best type of exercise is ongoing participation. Aerobic exercise is key, but even better outcomes occur when you combine aerobic exercise, resistance training, and flexibility training with mental exercise programs. We discussed mental exercise in Lecture 3 on self-care. The greatest effects on cognition seem to occur when exercise sessions exceed 30 minutes per session. Exercise influences executive control in particular, such as planning, scheduling, working memory, and task coordination.

As you get older, as you have more aches and pains, on those days when you're tired and you hurt and you just want to stay in bed and feel sorry for yourself, think about whether that's really in your best interest. I can tell you from direct experience with more than one family member and more than one student in my fitness classes that one decision to stay in bed one morning because it hurt too much to get up can snowball into a couple of days in bed, which snowballs to a week, which can lead to a chain reaction. When that happened, those individuals never got out of bed again.

My mother has severe chronic pain, from multiple chronic conditions: arthritis, fibromyalgia, severe osteoporosis, degeneration of her spine, sciatica, diabetic nerve pain, but she gets out of bed every morning at 6 am in spite of it, and she doesn't take any pain medication, because she is determined to use mind over matter to keep moving and stay active and engaged. That's what I'm encouraging you to do—to push through it and stay active. We should also encourage our children and grandchildren to be active for the cognitive benefits. Even though many schools are so focused on test performance that they are cutting activities like physical education and recess, research has shown that children who regularly engage in physical activity actually perform better in the classroom, including on standardized tests.

That benefit for work and performance holds for adults as well: Exercise has been associated with improved work efficiency, reduced absenteeism from work, even reduced errors at work. Not only will you perform better at work if you exercise, you might even earn more. One study found that exercising three times a week was correlated with a 6–10 percent increase in wages. You could chalk it up to the idea that pretty people make more money, but the study also reported that the increase in pay held regardless of body mass index—so it wasn't the way these individuals looked in their suits that mattered, it was the fact that they were going to the gym, working out regularly. Even participants who only worked out three times a month, barely once a week, still made five percent more income than their completely sedentary peers.

In contrast, another research study found that obese women earned 18 percent less than normal weight women, and a third study found that overweight women have a total family income of 25 percent less than normal weight women. So the health costs of not exercising are profound because now, not only do you have the extra costs of the health impacts of not exercising, you may actually earn less if you don't exercise.

Exercise is also powerful for promoting psychological health. Regular exercise helps to reduce stress, anxiety, anger, and depression, and reduces your risk level for developing clinical anxiety and depression. In fact, exercise can reduce symptoms of clinical depression in older adults by as much as 88 percent. Adults who are inactive are more likely to be depressed. Overall, the National Institute of Mental Health has concluded: Physical fitness is positively associated with mental health and well-being; that exercise specifically helps reduce stress and anxiety; that exercise helps reduce mild to moderate depression; and that even in severe cases of clinical anxiety and depression, exercise is a useful adjunct to psychotherapy and other forms of clinical treatment.

Interestingly, research studies on the impact of exercise on anxiety and depression have found that while more exercise has more impact, any exercise at all can help improve mood. There may be differences in how much of an impact based on the type, intensity, and duration of the exercise program, but any exercise at all of any kind will improve your mood. In fact, for day-to-day mood, research has found that regardless of how many negative or positive events you experienced in a single day, doing a single exercise session will improve your mood!

Nine weeks may be the sweet spot for more substantive benefits—nine weeks of regular exercise seems to be the point at which patients experience significant effective outcomes in reducing depression. In fact, a longer-term exercise program can be as effective as psychotherapy or medication in treating depression. The nice part is, long-term studies have shown that reductions in anxiety are not connected to the physical changes of fitness levels. Even if you don't feel like you're getting more fit, even if you're not losing weight, exercise will still have a positive impact on your mood.

There are other benefits of exercise; for instance, regular exercise has been demonstrated to improve life satisfaction, increasing your sense of positive affect, promoting overall well-being, promoting, quality of life, improve your sense of self, including a more positive self-concept, improved body image, higher self-esteem, and a greater sense of self-efficacy, which is your belief in your ability to accomplish specific tasks.

Initially, researchers assumed that exercise led to improved self-confidence and self-esteem because it made you more fit. They thought that you looked better, so you felt better about yourself. Research shows that while some of the improved self-confidence is related to improved fitness levels, not all of it is, because even if you don't become significantly more fit, or lose much weight, exercise can still improve self-confidence and self-esteem. It may be related to the physiological effects on hormones which affect mood. The benefits may be related to a sense of accomplishment and achievement. It could also be related to improved internal locus of control; as we talked about in Lecture 1, internal locus of control is related to a greater sense of control over your environment and a greater capacity to control your health, your well-being, and other outcomes. Exercise has been found to increase internal locus of control.

What exercise program is most likely to promote psychological health? Research has identified some key components. First, the exercise program needs to include rhythmic, abdominal breathing. Aerobic exercises like swimming and walking inherently do this; you breathe rhythmically as you do aerobic activity, but so can mindful fitness practices such as yoga and Tai Chi. Second, the exercise program needs to provide a relative absence of interpersonal competition. Competition can be fun; it can be exciting for some people, but it can also lead to overtraining, pressure to win, and a sense of social evaluation (which the idea that others are judging your performance). Research shows that noncompetitive forms of exercise are most likely to promote psychological health.

But the idea of noncompetitive exercise is not as clear-cut as you might think. You can run marathons or compete in triathlons with a noncompetitive mindset, where you are working only to complete your personal best. My chiropractor regularly does triathlons to stay fit as he gets older, but his focus is on his own time and performance. He's competing with himself, not with other people. In contrast, I have had yoga students who spent their time looking around the class to see who's doing the "best" warrior pose and who's doing the "deepest" backbend, who's the most flexible. Through their perspective, they turned something that should be mindful and internally focused into a competition with others. Your own mindset is key to whether or not there is the relative absence of interpersonal competition. If you find yourself at the gym trying to run faster than the person on the treadmill next to you, take a pause and reflect on who you're really competing with and why.

Third, exercise that is done in a closed and predictable environment is most likely to promote psychological health. Again, mindset is key here. For someone who is comfortable swimming, a pool is a closed environment: You know what to expect. For someone who plays golf regularly, a golf course provides that same set of boundaries and established expectations. Even trail hiking or mountain climbing can be closed environments if you do them regularly and are comfortable in the environment. The key is that generally speaking, self-paced environments where you have a good set of expectations for what the environment holds provide a safe, predictable environment so that you can focus on the activity, without distraction, allowing for more enjoyment of the activity itself.

Fourth, while, as we discussed, any exercise will promote some mental health benefits, to experience consistent improvement in well-being, you need to exercise for at least 20 minutes a day, at least two to three times per week. You'll notice that the amount of exercise you need to promote mental health is actually less than what you need for physical health. For physical health, you need at least 30 minutes—it can be broken up into three 10-minute blocks—at least five days per week. So, if you're doing enough exercise to keep your physical heart ticking healthfully, you're also doing enough exercise to keep your emotional heart feeling loved and loving.

Finally, the most critical component of an exercise program intended to promote psychological health may be the most obvious thing you're unlikely to think of. You need to enjoy it. We often associate exercise with something we just put on our to-do list and slog through. If you find an exercise program you truly enjoy, you're more likely both to do it, and to benefit from it. We talked about different types of exercise in Lecture 5, Fitness Outside the Gym, and we'll talk more about our psychological need for fun in our final lecture.

Pull out your journal. For today's takeaway, think through everything we've talked about. What are the health characteristics you want to promote? Heart health? Brain health? Strength and the ability to carry your own groceries? Stress management? There are no wrong reasons; they are all good, valid answers and valid reasons to get fit. So identify your health reasons, the personal health needs that will inspire you to keep going. Focus on framing your motivators in a positive context rather than a negative one, stating "I want to have a healthy heart" rather than "I want to avoid a heart attack." It may not seem like a big difference, but the positive framework of what you're trying to achieve, instead of what you're trying to avoid, can lead to better outcomes.

Reflect on your experience with this course so far. What benefits have you already experienced from exercise? Then, assess your own level of competitiveness. When, where, how do you compete against others? Do you rush to get in line first at the grocery store? Do you rush to talk first in a meeting? Do you always make the decision about where you will eat with friends or what movie you'll see?

If so, what's your internal motivation for that feeling of competition? Are you afraid of looking bad? Are you afraid of being left out? Are you afraid of missing something? How does that affect your fitness? Is fear of "not winning" keeping you from trying something new, because you might be awkward or embarrassed? Think about how many times you've missed out on something because your internal sense of competition made you afraid you might lose. Ask yourself: What is it that you might lose? What can you do to better support yourself in giving up that inner urge for competition, so that you can be more open and try more things that are new and enjoy them just for the sake of enjoyment?

With all these benefits of exercise—benefits for your physical health, for your psychological health, for your cognitive functioning—the big question is, why don't we all do it? Take a moment, and try to think of one other single activity that could so completely affect your health, across the board. I can't think of anything else that has so much potential for good. And all it requires is 150 minutes a week. Just two-and-a-half hours. We spend 13 hours a week sending emails, and those don't provide that kind of positive impact on our health, well-being, and quality of life. In fact, research has shown that all sorts of other variables—income, education, marital status, age—are not significantly related to perceptions of quality of life. But exercise is. Such a simple thing, something totally within your control, and it can truly improve your life.

Making It Work—The Right Plan for You
Lecture 12

For children, physical activity and movement are related to fun and independence. As they become older, we encourage children to engage in physical activity to get good grades in gym class, to build character, and even to earn scholarships to college. Later in life, we come to understand that exercise is good for our health and will help prevent disease, and while that's true, the problem with looking at exercise as something that leads to an outcome is that we start to perceive it as work or an obligation. In this lecture, we'll look at intrinsic motivations for participating in physical activities.

Self-Determination Theory

- Self-determination theory proposes that we have three innate psychological needs: competence, autonomy, and relatedness. We are motivated by things that support fulfillment of these three needs. They provide internal—intrinsic—motivation to participate in activities. External—extrinsic—factors can motivate you in the short term, but in the long run, extrinsic factors can actually reduce your motivation.

- This idea is contrary to our perceptions of how to promote behavior. We grow up with the idea that extrinsic rewards motivate us. If we do well in school, we get good grades. If we do well at work, we get pay raises and promotions. But those kinds of extrinsic rewards work only in limited settings and conditions, and sometimes, even the most seemingly innocent of external rewards can reduce motivation.

- Self-determination theory holds that we have a deep, internal need to feel as if we are competent, that is, good at what we do; autonomous, that we are masters of our own universe; and related—connected to others. To really make exercise fit into our lives, we need to choose activities that make us feel good about ourselves, that we choose for ourselves, and that reinforce our relationships.

Making Exercise Habitual

- Large portions of our lives are habitual; about 45% of everyday activities are repeated in the same way and the same location almost every day. Many of us never skip such healthy habits as flossing and brushing our teeth.

- However, it can be challenging to turn exercise into a habit. Exercise is a habit for only 22% of the population, while 54% of the population exercises occasionally but not enough for the practice to be considered a habit. Engaging in occasional exercise makes it more difficult to experience any benefits. Most people who begin a new exercise program stick to it for only about 5 weeks before they lapse.

- One aspect that affects habit is having a stable environment. You brush your teeth at your bathroom sink, not outside at the garden house or in the kitchen. The consistency of location and availability of your toothbrush and toothpaste make it easy and simple to brush your teeth. The tools and the location both support your habit. Consider how you can provide a similarly consistent environment for exercise behaviors.
  - For example, keep your walking shoes by the door so that you don't have to search for them when you want to go for a walk. Better yet, keep one pair of walking shoes in your desk at work and one in your car to take advantage of other opportunities to walk that may arise throughout the day. Keep a yoga mat on the floor beside your bed so that you can do 10 minutes of stretching to relax and unwind before you go to bed.

  - Also make sure you wear clothes that promote movement. Wear flats instead of high heels so that you can take the stairs instead of the elevator.

- ○ Set up your treadmill, stationary bike, or elliptical machine in front of a TV so that you can get a workout while you watch.

- The ways in which you structure your environment must be connected to your intrinsic motivation for exercise and fitness. You want the environmental structure to promote your internal motivation for exercising—to connect to your philosophical needs for competence, autonomy, and relatedness. Setting up your environment in a way that makes exercise feel like an obligation will actually reduce your motivation.

Finding the Joy in Exercise

- Probably the most powerful reason you'll find to exercise is that it's fun. You will be most likely to commit to fitness throughout your lifetime if you find a type of fitness activity that you enjoy. Don't go to the gym and slog through a workout you hate. Don't exercise because your doctor tells you to or you think you should. Find an activity you truly enjoy that makes you want to engage it.

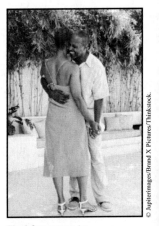

- If you haven't found this activity yet, keep trying new and different things until you do. Even fitness instructors don't necessarily like to take fitness classes, such as aerobics. You may find that you enjoy hiking with your family, exploring your city on foot, swimming, dancing, or practicing yoga or Tai Chi.

Find fun ways to incorporate fitness "moments" into your everyday life, such as playing chase with your children or dancing with your spouse.

- As mentioned in an earlier lecture, preconceived notions about your athletic ability can serve as barriers to fitness change. Don't cling to labels, such as "bookworm," that were placed on you when you were young. What you were as a child doesn't have to define you now. Take control of your health and choose to age healthfully and with enjoyment.

- An interesting research approach compared a focus on "hoped-for selves"—the selves we hope to be and maintain, such as healthy and independent—with a focus on "feared selves"—the selves we are afraid of and want to avoid, such as unhealthy and dependent.
  ○ The older adults who used the hoped-for selves approach had improved positive self-perception and higher levels of exercise and exercise adherence.

  ○ Focus on the positive outcome—on healthy aging—and then make decisions to get there. Above it all, figure out how to make those decisions and the journey to your hoped-for self fun.

Reaching a Healthy Lifestyle

- In this course, we've talked about many different theories of motivation and different strategies for promoting fitness success. Let's look at what might be the best approach to getting you to a healthy lifestyle.

- First, you have to have a positive outlook. Think about what you want to be—that hoped-for self—instead of what you want to avoid. Identify the healthy aging you want to have and focus your eyes on that horizon so that you're driving toward that goal.

- Second, set goals that you can buy into. Identify a philosophical vision of who you are and who you want to be. In doing this, you should think about the basic needs outlined in self-determination theory—competence, autonomy, and relatedness—and figure out how your fitness plan can fulfill those needs. Identify the motivations that are rewards in themselves, such as a feeling of energy, happiness, and connectedness with family and friends, so that exercise becomes intrinsically motivated.

- Third, turn your positive approach and your philosophical vision into concrete action by setting SMART goals about the steps that will help you achieve your vision. The vision is the what and the why, and the SMART goals are the how. Keep in mind that if your actionable goals are connected to things you find fun and truly enjoy, you're much more likely to achieve them. Don't allow your inner parent to push you so much that fitness stops being fun and you quit; instead, nurture your inner child with fitness activities that bring joy.

- Fourth, set up your environment to support your success in a way that feels good, not obligatory. Life is hard enough; make fitness an easy choice. Have the tools and the equipment you need on hand. Put fitness on your calendar and consider it a reward to yourself for accomplishing the other things you have to do.

- Fifth, keep track—not to punish yourself but to remind yourself of what matters, of what you value. Keep yourself accountable to your philosophical vision of your hoped-for self. It's easy to get so caught up in chores, to-do lists, emails, and deadlines that you lose track of what you really believe in. Prioritize the things that matter to you and put first things first. Maintain the journal you started in this course and use it to keep yourself accountable to your vision of healthy aging. That physical reminder of your success will make you feel even better about yourself, and your satisfaction will lead to even more success.

- Finally, remember that fitness is a journey—an ongoing process.
  - Periodically, you'll need to reset your SMART goals. Maybe you'll get injured and have to start over. Maybe an activity you enjoy will stop being fun, or the yoga teacher you love will move away, or the pool you swim in will close. Life might get in the way, and your fitness may fall by the wayside for a time. Don't beat yourself up if that happens; just pick yourself up and start again.

- o   Even if you stay committed and keep going, you should still plan to assess your motivations and goals. Pick a time to build this assessment into your life, perhaps at the start of each season or on your birthday. Reevaluate where you are, where you want to be, and how you're going to get there. And always keep in mind that the best exercise program is the one you actually do.

Suggested Reading

Deci and Flaste, *Why We Do What We Do*.

Pink, *Drive*.

Activities and Assignments

Reflect on your environment—your home and office, your schedule, and the time and space requirements of your life. Identify unique challenges and support systems in this environment and find strategies for addressing them to make your environment stable and supportive of fitness. How can you better structure your environment to make exercise a healthy habit that is easy to keep? Even more important, how can you structure those environmental cues in a meaningful way that connects to your deeper internal motivation for exercise?

Go back to your fitness plan from Lecture 4. Is it still working for you? How does it make you feel? Are you experiencing the fitness gains you hoped for? Do you enjoy the activities you've chosen or do they feel like a chore? Where do you need to make modifications? Is it time to increase intensity, duration, or frequency? Is it time to change modality? Update your fitness plan as needed and make sure it will help you achieve your goals while having fun.

Go back to the SMART goals from Lecture 7. How are you doing with your goals? Are you still working on them? Do you need to revise them or set new ones? Update your SMART goals as needed and make sure they support your positive view of healthy aging and your vision of your hoped-for self.

Establish a plan for keeping yourself accountable. How will you keep track so that you can prioritize what matters? Identify a journal, a calendar, or even a technology tool to help you focus on your priorities.

Set a date for yourself for when you will revisit your fitness plan, your SMART goals, and your strategies for accountability. Set the goal for at least 6 weeks from when you start a fitness program, so that you have a chance to turn your healthy activities into habits.

Making It Work—The Right Plan for You
Lecture 12—Transcript

Over 50 million children play sports. Parents may encourage their children to play sports because of the perceived direct and indirect benefits; for instance, the notion that sport participation builds character and develops leadership skills. Many parents also anticipate sport scholarships to help with college, and hope their children will have professional careers as athletes. The reality? Research is inconsistent about the character-building impact of sports. Sports don't teach character. Adults teach character, and if the adults who coach and lead a child's sports team encourage winning above teamwork and ethical behavior, then sports will promote bad character traits, not good ones. The professional career is a long shot. Of those high school seniors who are varsity athletes, less than 1 percent will end up playing professionally. And those scholarships? Also rare. Among high school seniors who are varsity athletes, only 2.9 percent will go on to play basketball at an NCAA college, and only 5.6 percent of the baseball and football players will end up on NCAA rosters. Even fewer are on athletic scholarships, with between 1 and 2 percent of undergraduate students receiving an athletic scholarship, depending on the year. In contrast, two-thirds of fulltime undergraduate students have some combination of assistance from need-based grants and merit-based scholarships. *U.S. News and World Report* indicates that at colleges who focus on merit-based scholarships, the percentage of fulltime undergraduates on academic scholarships can range from 27 percent up to 88 percent!

We get it wrong from day one. We teach our kids to do sports to earn a grade in PE or earn a scholarship or learn character. But none of those reasons will sustain fitness throughout the lifespan. In fact, among kids, 70 percent quit playing sports before they even get to high school. The number one reason why kids quit sports? It stops being fun. A toddler learning to walk doesn't run across the house to learn something or achieve something; he runs for the sheer joy of running. The sheer joy of being able to control his body, learn how to move, and be independent. Think about how hard small children work just to get the right to move. My son is two years younger than my daughter is, and it has been fascinating watching his determination to move as fast and as well as she does, just so that he can keep up with all the fun his big sister is having.

Here's a very interesting contrast. Perhaps you've heard of using a pedometer to track your steps throughout the day. We talked about it earlier in the course. To do this, you clip a pedometer on your waistline as soon as you get up in the morning, and you let it count every step you take until you go to bed at night. As we talked about, a good goal is to accumulate 10,000 steps in a day. At an average adult gait, that's about 5 miles of walking. If you focus on being active throughout your day, and also add in 30 to 60 minutes of deliberate walking, you will likely achieve 10,000 steps. But most people fall short. Various research studies indicate that the average America active adult takes between 5,100 and 6,500 steps per day. Inactive adults take less than 3,000 steps per day.

In contrast, the average toddler—a new walker between the ages of one and two—takes 2,368 steps per hour! Over the course of a day, the average toddler takes more than 14,000 steps, enough steps for those little feet to walk across 46 football fields. Granted, a toddler's 14,000 steps are meandering, stop and look out the window at a flower, then pick up a block, then run to mommy's legs kinds of walks, but still, far more movement than we do as adults. So movement starts out about fun and independence and the pure joy of it.

And then we're told that we should do it, that it's good for us, that we have to meet presidential fitness standards in PE class, and earn a passing grade. We're told it will build our character and help us get to college. Later, we're told it's good for our health, and it will help prevent disease. And while all of those disease-fighting characteristics we talked about in our last lecture on the benefits of physical activity are true, the problem with looking at exercise as something that leads to an outcome is that we start to look at exercise as work, as an obligation.

We talked about goal setting in motivation part 2, and goal setting is important in supporting you in achieving the outcomes you desire. As we discussed, you are more able to stay on track and achieve goals that are SMART Specific, Measurable, Attainable, Realistic, and Time-Specific. But, as humans, we also have an innate need for meaning, and research shows that we actually prefer goals that are enduring and abstract, so that we can philosophically commit to them. So there is some irony and contradiction here: We feel better and more committed to goals like "I am a good mother" and "I am a fit and healthy person," but we are more likely to achieve a goal like "I will read to my children every night before bed for 15 minutes" and "I will go for a 30-minute walk three days a week." So we need to set specific SMART goals to support us in achieving them, but they need to be framed in an overall philosophical context that we can connect to, and which gives our goals a greater purpose.

Self-determination theory proposes that we have three innate psychological needs: competence, autonomy, and relatedness We are motivated by things that support fulfillment of these three needs. They provide the internal, the intrinsic motivation to participate in activities. When you let external or extrinsic factors motivate you, it can work in the short term, but in the long term, it can actually reduce your motivation. If you're afraid of a health condition and your doctor tells you that you "should" exercise, you might do it for a while. Your doctor, an expert told you that you should. But over the long run should doesn't work. Extrinsic motivators don't work in the long run.

This can turn your whole view of motivation and human behavior upside down because it's contrary to our perceptions of how to promote behavior. We grow up with the idea that extrinsic rewards motivate us. If we do well in school we get gold stars and then we get As on our report card. If we do well at work, we get pay raises and promotions. But those kinds of extrinsic rewards only work in certain settings and in limited conditions and sometimes even the most seemingly innocent of external rewards can actually reduce motivation.

Let me give you a research example. There was a research study with children who loved to draw and who used their free playtime to draw. Researchers divided the children into three groups. The first group were given expectations of an award: They were showed a certificate and a blue ribbon, and told that if they drew they would receive the award. The second group were asked if they wanted to draw, and if they drew, then at the end of the session, they were given the award. The third group was just provided the opportunity to draw with no award and no discussion of awards. Two weeks later, the children were observed during free playtime. The surprise-award and the no-award group were still drawing for fun. But the expected-award group showed less interest and spent less time drawing. So something that was fun and intrinsically motivated was actually ruined by the introduction of extrinsic motivators.

So, self-determination theory holds that we have a deep, internal need to feel like we are competent—good at what we do—that we are autonomous, masters of our own universe; and that we are related, connected to others. So to really make exercise fit into your life, you need to pick something that makes you feel good about yourself, pick something that you choose for yourself, and ideally, pick something that reinforces your relationships.

You might also be able to help exercise fit into your life if it is habitual. In fact, large portions of our lives are habitual: About 45 percent of everyday activities are repeated in the same way and the same location almost every day. Think about some habits that you have that are health promoting. What are the healthy habits that you never skip, precisely because you never skip them, so you don't even think of it as an option? Every night, no matter what, I wash my face, floss, brush my teeth, and rinse with mouthwash. No matter how sick I am, how tired, whatever, I do those things. Always. It's challenging, though, to turn a habit like exercise into a habit like brushing your teeth. Only 22 percent of the population successfully turn exercise into a habit and do it regularly. Fifty-four percent of the population exercise occasionally, but not enough for it to be a habit, which makes it that much harder for them to do it enough to experience any benefits. In fact, most people who begin a new exercise program only stick to it for about five weeks before they lapse.

One aspect that affects habit is having a stable environment. You brush your teeth at your bathroom sink every night. You probably don't brush them at the outside garden house or the kitchen sink. So the consistency of location and the easy availability of your toothbrush and toothpaste make it simple to brush your teeth. The tools and the location both support your habit.

So think about: How can you do the same for exercise? How can you make the environment stable, so that the location, the tools, and the environmental cues all support your exercise behaviors? Keep your walking shoes right by the back door, so it's easy to put them on and go for a walk. Maybe you even have three pairs of walking shoes: one in your desk at work, so that you can take a quick walk at lunch; one you keep in your car, so you can go for walk instead of just waiting in the car when your kids are in an activity or you're picking them up from school; one pair by your back door to make a walk after dinner with your spouse easy. Maybe you can keep a yoga mat on the floor beside your bed, so that it's easy to do 10 minutes of stretching right before you go to bed to relax and unwind. Also think about clothes that promote movement.

Let me give you a personal example about my clothing decisions: I very rarely wear high heels. I wear flat, comfortable shoes because for me in comfortable shoes, I can take the stairs instead of the elevator. I can walk around the block if I've got 15 minutes free. During a break between meetings, I can do a couple of stretches to wake up. There's a lot you can do, when your clothes don't get in the way.

Think that way about things you could do in your home or space that would work for you. My husband loves action movies, and I'm not a big fan. He set up his elliptical in front of a TV, so he watches movies while he does his cardio. He always plans to do an hour, but sometimes he does more, an hour and a half, two hours, because the movie gets good and he doesn't want to stop midway through. So maybe that would work for you, and as long as it makes you happy, who cares if you have a treadmill or a stationary bike or an elliptical in your living room? It's better than having one in a storage room just gathering dust. Think outside the box, be OK with making decisions that promote your health, even if they seem unconventional to other people.

But here is the kicker about your environment: The ways in which you structure your environment need to be connected to your intrinsic motivation for exercise and fitness. You want that environmental structure to promote your internal motivation for exercising, to connect to your philosophical need for competence, and autonomy, and relatedness. If you set your environment up in a way that exercise feels like an obligation, something you should do, something that is not autonomous but that's being forced on you by the environment, then it will actually lose the power of activation and it will not support you in facilitating exercise behavior.

So, as one takeaway activity for today, I'd like you to reflect on your own environment: your home, your office, your schedule, and the time and space requirements of your life. Identify your unique challenges and support systems. Then, think about strategies for how you can address those challenges to make your environment stable and supportive of your fitness. How can you better structure your environment to make exercise a healthy habit that is easy to keep? And, even more importantly, how can you structure those environmental cues in a meaningful way that connects to your deep internal motivation for exercise?

Let's go back now to that reason that kids play sports, and the reason why they quit. Fun, joy, because that's the most powerful reason you will find to exercise. You will be most likely to commit to fitness throughout your lifetime if you figure out how to enjoy it. Yes, you will get health benefits and you may live longer, but you're doing it because you enjoy the experience of it, because it helps you feel young, energized, and like you've regained a sense of adventure. What that means is finding a type of fitness you actually enjoy. Don't go to the gym and slog through a workout you hate. Don't do it because your doctor tells you to or you think you should or I told you to in this course. Find something you really enjoy.

If you haven't found it, keep trying new and different things until you do. I've encouraged you to build exercise as a habit, but I'd like you to build a habit around something that feels great for you. So keep trying new things until you find the ones that make you excited. Go back to Lecture, Fitness beyond the Gym, for inspiration. Watch little kids, your own or your grandkids or a friend's kids or kids at the park. Remember the things you did when you were young that made your heart sing. Spin in circles? Play hopscotch? Swing on the swings? Jump on a trampoline? Play stickball in the street? Find what you love

I have many fitness certifications, and I'm trained to teach group fitness classes like aerobics and step aerobics. But I don't enjoy taking those kinds of classes; to me, they feel repetitive, and I don't really like watching myself in the mirror, and they're so noisy that they make my head hurt. So I don't take them, and because of that I don't teach them. What I love to do is go for hikes with my family, and explore new neighborhoods or walk through a zoo or visit a new city or find a new country trail so I'm out walking. I love to swim laps, but only in a warm pool, because if the pool is cold, it makes my body hurt. I love the warm relaxed feeling and the mellow focus after I do Tai Chi or yoga. I love to dance, and if my husband and I can ever find a few minutes to do a salsa or a cha-cha, it leaves me feeling happier, and more energized, and more connected to my spouse for several hours after. So find what you love.

I have a family friend and she has a daughter who is playing sports in school. I asked her about her son, and if he was playing sports, and she said, "No, not really, he's kind of a bookworm." That resonated with me as something to think about because I was a bookworm. My mother was in the army and we moved all the time, so books were my best friends growing up. I was very small: I started the seventh grade at 4'9" and 72 pounds, which means I was about half the size of everyone else in my middle school. I was also extremely injury prone: I broke my wrist, I broke my ankle, I got bone bruises and sprains. So I wasn't fast, I wasn't strong, and I wasn't great at sports. I was picked last for teams every time they were picked in PE. I was absolutely terrified of the mile run because you had to run an eight-minute mile to just pass, and that stupid run threatened my straight-A report card every year of elementary school and middle school.

But, my family encouraged fitness in ways that I enjoyed, so we walked the dogs together, we went swimming regularly, I gardened with my grandma and grandpa, I took dance lessons and roller-skating lessons and tennis lessons, so I stayed fit, but I didn't think of myself as athletic. So, if you had told me when I was a kid that I would someday make a career out of teaching others about exercise and fitness, I wouldn't have believed you, because I wasn't an athlete. I was a sickly kid who was allergic to everything and caught every bug that came my way. My immune system was so fragile that I got shingles at 15. I challenge you to find anyone else who has gotten shingles as a child. I still struggle with a variety of stress-related health conditions: allergies, eczema, high cholesterol, and some chronic pain. But my point is that here

I am. And maybe the fact that I am is proof that anyone can take control of their health and choose to age healthfully. We label our kids so young; we say they're bookworms or they're jocks or they're whatever, but break your labels and write new ones. Who you were as a kid doesn't have to define you now. Find your joy.

So what if I wasn't an athlete at 7 or 12 or 17. So what if I was a sickly kid. I'm strong, fit, and healthy now. When my daughter throws me a ball I throw it back because it's fun, and she giggles. When my son kicks a ball I kick it back to him and we laugh and play and run around the room. I still don't like running, but when my daughter says, "Mama, chase me" I run after her and have so much fun playing chase, that I forget that I'm even running and then we collapse and giggle and have a really good time.

So maybe you were a bookworm, too; well, then be smart enough to value fitness and to be able to explore options until you find something you enjoy. Maybe you were picked last in PE class. Maybe you were a jock and earned your letter jacket and then were surprised when you didn't get a big college scholarship and then go off to play sports professionally. But so what? Who we were as kids doesn't matter now. Those labels we had, we don't have to keep them. We can all be athletes. We can all be fit. We can all enjoy exercise. What matters is that you're not sitting on the bench now. And if you are still on the bench, 12 lectures into this course, then what matters is that you decide to stand up, and get moving.

An interesting research approach compared a focus on "hoped-for selves," in other words, the things you hope to be and maintain, such as staying healthy and independent, with a focus on "feared selves," the things you are afraid of and want to avoid, such as avoiding negative health outcomes or dependence. The older adults who used the hoped-for selves approach had improved positive self-perception and higher levels of exercise and exercise adherence. So it goes back to the optimism of our centenarians. Focus on the hopeful, on the positive outcome, on the healthy aging you want to live, and then make decisions to help you get there. And above it all, figure out how to make those decisions, and that journey to your hoped-for self, fun.

As we come to the end of our course, what's the bottom line? We've talked about many different theories of motivation, and different strategies for promoting your fitness success. Let me offer what I see as the best approach to get you to a healthy lifestyle. First, you have to use a positive approach: Think about what you want to be, that hoped-for self, instead of what you want to avoid. You're identifying the healthy aging that you want to have, and then focusing your eyes on that horizon, so that you are driving towards what you want. Like our centenarians, you're being optimistic.

Second, you need to set goals that you can buy into. You need to identify a philosophical vision of who you are, and who you want to be. In doing this, you should think about the basic needs as outlined in self-determination theory: competence, autonomy, and relatedness, and figure out how your fitness plan can fulfill those needs. Identify the motivations that are rewards in themselves—feeling energetic, feeling happy, feeling connected with your family and friends—so that exercise becomes intrinsically motivated.

Third, turn your positive approach and your philosophical vision into concrete action by setting SMART goals about the steps that will help you to achieve your vision. The vision is the so what, and the why; the SMART goals are the how. Remember that if your actionable goals are connected to things you find fun and truly enjoy, you're much more likely to achieve them. Don't allow your inner parent to push you so much that fitness stops being fun and you quit; instead, nurture your inner child with fitness activities that bring joy.

Fourth, set up your environment to support your success, in a way that feels good, not obligatory. Life is hard enough; make fitness an easy choice. Have the tools and the equipment on hand that you need. Put it on your calendar and look at it as a reward to yourself for accomplishing the other things you have to do. It's self-care so that you take care of yourself and your well-being for the long haul.

Fifth, keep track. Not to punish yourself, but to remind yourself of what matters, and of what you value. Keep yourself accountable to your philosophical vision of your hoped-for self. It's so easy to just let life run over you. To get so caught up in the chores and the to-do lists and the emails that you lose track of what you really believe in. Unless you're a brain surgeon or an emergency-room doctor, very few things are actually life or death. So prioritize the things that matter to you, and put first things first.

This is a place where I absolutely practice what I preach. I keep track, on a family calendar, of when I exercise. I write down when I do yoga, when I swim, when I go for a walk. But I don't just keep track of when I exercise, I keep track of everything that I feel matters to my well-being. I write down when I take my kids to the park. When we go to church. When we go on a family vacation, or a day trip to the zoo. When I have a date with my husband. Those are all things that I value, things that I think are important for my well-being, and the well-being of my family. And putting them on the calendar helps me remember that they are just as important as the doctor appointments and the work meetings. I don't want to let what seems urgent or required get in the way of what really matters to me.

So I encourage you to keep the journal you started with this course, and use it to keep track. Use it to keep yourself accountable to your heart and your vision of healthy aging. As you see that visual reminder of your success, you'll feel even better about yourself, and that satisfaction will lead to more success.

Sixth, and finally, remember that it's a journey. It's an ongoing process. You'll need to reset SMART goals periodically. Maybe you'll get injured and have to start over. Maybe an activity you enjoy will stop being fun, or the yoga teacher you love will move away, or the pool you swim in will close. Life might get in the way, urgent things will overcome you, and your fitness will fall by the wayside. It's OK. Don't beat yourself up. Pick yourself up, dust off your knees, and get back on the horse.

Maybe you will stay committed, and you'll keep going, and life won't get in the way, but you should still make a plan to regularly assess your motivations and your goals. Pick a time to build this into your life, perhaps the start of each season, or on your birthday once a year, or at New Year's if you like to do resolutions and sweep out the cobwebs as you start a new year. What matters is that you deliberately make the effort to regularly assess where you are, where you want to be, and how you're going to get there.

It's time for our takeaways, so pull out your trusty journal. First, do the exercise we discussed earlier in this lecture: Reflect on your environment, your challenges, and how you can structure your environment to support your success. Now, let's assess what we've done so far in this course, and how we will keep you on track. Go back to FITT plan you built in the fitness fundamentals lecture. Is it still working for you? How does it make you feel? Are you experiencing the fitness gains you hoped for? Do you enjoy it or does it feel like a chore? Where do you need to make modifications? Perhaps it's to increase intensity, time or frequency. Perhaps it's time to try a new type of exercise. Update your fitness plan as needed, and make sure it will help you achieve your goals and help you have fun.

Now, go back to the SMART goals you set in the motivation part 2 lecture. How are you doing with them? Are you still working on them? Do you need to revise them, or perhaps set new ones? Update your SMART goals as needed, and make sure they support your positive view of healthy aging, and your vision of your hoped-for self.

Finally, set a plan for keeping yourself accountable—how will you keep track, so that you prioritize what matters. Identify a journal, or a calendar, or even a technology tool, to help you keep your focus on your priorities. Set a date for yourself for when you will revisit your fitness plan, your SMART goals, and your strategies for accountability. Set the goal for at least six weeks from today, so that you have a good chance to turn your healthy activities into a healthy habit.

I hope that, through this course, I've helped you to learn more about exercise and fitness, and how to fit them into your life, and what a difference it can make once you do. I also hope I've opened your eyes to many options for building fitness and activity into your life. There are so many ways that you can stay active, that you can support your fitness, and they all promote healthy aging, so pick the one that you love and that brings you joy—because at the end of the day, the best exercise routine is the one you actually do.

Relaxation Strategies
Lecture 13

In this lecture, we will go through four relaxation techniques: 15 minutes of progressive relaxation, 5 minutes of meditation using the anapana breathing technique, 5 minutes of meditation using alternate nostril breathing, and a 5-minute Reiki energy session. As you'll see, these techniques can be used at any time to relieve stress, help you learn to control your thoughts, energize you, or provide relief from pain.

Progressive Relaxation

- Progressive relaxation is a relaxation technique based on contracting your muscles. It can be helpful for learning to recognize what muscular tension feels like. Indeed, you may find that you carry around more residual tension than you realize. This technique can also be helpful for dealing with insomnia; if you try it while lying down in bed at night, you may find that you fall asleep more easily and sleep more deeply.

- In this session, we'll do a full-body progressive relaxation exercise, but you can also do only a partial exercise if you need a quick stress management strategy. For instance, if you're at work and feeling tense, you might do an abbreviated series focusing on your upper body, neck, and back.

- Because this technique involves isometric contractions, if you have high blood pressure or a history of heart disease, please consult your doctor before trying progressive relaxation. Also, be aware that as you contract your muscles, you might get a muscle cramp or spasm, particularly the first time you try the technique. This is normal; if you experience any cramping, just move the limb gently.

- For this session, we'll work through the entire body with a series of contractions and releases. If possible, lie down flat on your back on your bed or on an exercise mat on the floor. You can use a pillow under your head; if you have lower back issues, place a pillow or bolster under your knees to keep your lower back more comfortable.

- We will start with the toes and work our way up the body, contracting and releasing the muscles in the feet, legs, abdomen, and so on. At the end of the exercise, we'll contract and release all the muscles in the body, and you will feel yourself becoming heavy, sinking into the floor or bed beneath you. Try to hold onto this sense of complete relaxation.

Anapana Sati
- Anapana sati, the meditation on in-and-out breathing, is a simple exercise to help you focus your awareness and learn deliberate control of your thoughts. In anapana sati meditation, you use the sensation of your breath as an anchor for your focus.

- For this technique, begin in a comfortable seated position. You can sit in a chair, or if you're comfortable sitting on the floor in a cross-legged or kneeling position, you can use that position. The key is that your posture should be soft and relaxed; you should not be distracted by discomfort.

- During this meditation, focus your awareness on the physical sensation of your breath—breathing in and out through the nose. If your mind wanders, bring your awareness back to your nose and the way your breath feels as it flows in and out of your nostrils.

- This sensation-based meditation can bring you back to the present moment and your actual experience. You can practice it regularly to improve your ability to be centered in the moment, and you can use it as a tool during moments of stress.

Alternate Nostril Breathing
- Alternate nostril breathing is a yoga breathing technique that is wonderful for increasing your energy level. If you're feeling tired or fatigued or experiencing a headache or congestion, alternate nostril breathing can be a good technique to clear your mind.

- Because this breathing technique crosses the midline of the body, yoga theory also holds that it helps connect the right and left sides of the brain; this connection can be useful when you are faced with a task that requires both creative and analytical skills.

- Again, begin in a comfortable seated position. Your posture should be soft and relaxed so that you are not distracted by discomfort. You will inhale and exhale at the same time that you alternate closing one nostril and then the other.

- Alternate nostril breathing should leave you with a sense of being calm and energized, focused and awake. Set an intention to maintain this sense of calm, peaceful energy throughout the rest of your day.

Reiki Energy
- Reiki is a Japanese energy-based system that helps you to channel the warmth and energy of your body into your own healing. We'll

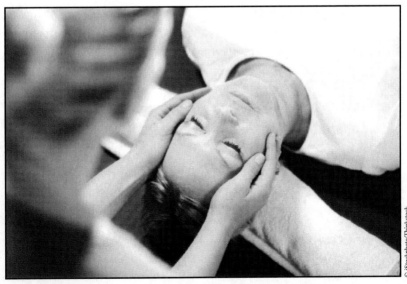

A brief Reiki session may reduce your anxiety about pain, making it seem more manageable.

do a brief Reiki session to help you learn how this technique can help you relax and work through pain or discomfort.

- In this technique, you first breathe into the palms of your hands. You then place your hands gently on a part of your body that may be injured or in pain. As you take deep, slow, deliberate breaths, think about that part of your body, imagining red blood cells rushing in with energy, white blood cells rushing in to heal, and your body connecting to its capacity to heal and repair itself.

- You can do this exercise at any time, focusing on any part of your body. It may not eliminate chronic pain, but it can reduce your perception and fear of pain, making the pain seem more manageable and helping you to feel in control of your thoughts and your body.

- You can also try this Reiki technique to support a loved one who needs loving energy and a compassionate touch.

Suggested Reading

Benson, *The Relaxation Response*.

Hart, *The Art of Living*.

Iynegar, *Light on Pranayama*.

Stein, *Essential Reiki*.

Vipassana Meditation, http://www.dhamma.org/.

Relaxation Strategies
Lecture 13—Transcript

Progressive Relaxation (15 minutes)

Progressive relaxation is a relaxation strategy based on contracting your muscles. It can be very helpful for learning to recognize what muscular tension feels like. You may find that you carry around more residual tension than you realize. Progressive relaxation is a helpful strategy for dealing with insomnia. If you try it while lying down in bed at night, you may find that you fall asleep more easily and sleep more deeply.

In this session, we'll do a full-body progressive relaxation exercise, but you can also do only a partial exercise if you need a quick stress-management strategy. For instance, if you're at work and feeling stressed and tense, you could do a quick series focusing on your upper body, neck and back. Because we will be using isometric contractions, if you have high blood pressure or a history of heart disease, please consult with your doctor prior to trying this relaxation strategy.

Also, be aware that as you contract your muscles, you might get a muscle cramp or spasm, particularly the first time you try progressive relaxation. This is normal, and if you experience any cramping, just move the limb gently. As we do contractions of the torso and abdomen, you may also experience some intestinal gas.

For this session, we'll work through your entire body with a series of contractions and releases. It's best to lie down flat on your back if possible, for instance on your bed or on an exercise mat on the floor. You can use a pillow under your head if you prefer. If you have low back issues, place a pillow or bolster under your knees to keep your low back more comfortable.

Lie down, in a comfortable position on the floor or bed. Feet are about hip width apart and relaxed outward. Arms are open gently at your sides, palms up. Close your eyes, and take a few deep breaths in and out through the nose. Breathe gently through your nose, with soft breaths into a relaxed belly.

We'll begin the progressive relaxation with your toes. Curl your right toes in and contract them gently. Hold the contraction as tight as you can. Remember to keep breathing. Relax your toes out completely. Contract your left toes. Hold tightly, remembering to breathe while you contract. Now release.

Now contract the toes of both the right and the left feet, contracting, holding that tension, feeling what tense feet feel like. Remember to continue breathing—it's easy to accidentally hold your breath. Then relax, release your feet out completely.

We'll move now to the calf of the right leg. Contract the muscle. Try to keep the foot relaxed and isolate the muscles in the calf of your right leg. Contract and hold it there, and then release it all the way out. Let's contract that muscle again. Contract the muscles of the right calf, hold it tight. And then release, all the way out. Let's take the left leg. Contract the muscles of the calf of the left leg. Hold tight, and then relax. Contract again, hold it there, and then release. Now let's talk both calves. Contract the right and the left. Hold tight, remember to breathe as you're tensing those muscles, and then release it out. One more time: Contract, and release.

Now let's move to the thighs. We'll start with the right thigh, and try to isolate the muscles of the thigh, keeping the lower leg and the foot relaxed. Clench the muscles of your right thigh, contract there and hold. Remember to breathe as you're contracting, and then release. Let's take the right thigh again; contract and hold, and then release. Now let's take the left thigh, again isolating the thigh muscles—keep the calf and the foot relaxed, contract the left thigh and hold, and release. Take it again. Contract, and release. Now let's take both thighs—contract the muscles and hold. Remember to breathe. And then release. And then contract again and hold it there … and relax, release it out.

Let's move now to your bottom, and you're going to try to keep your legs soft and isolate the muscles of your bottom. You're going to contract and hold that, but again, try to keep your thighs, your calves, your feet relaxed. Contracting specifically the bottom, focus there. Contract and hold, and then release. And again, contract, and release, relax.

Now we're going to try the whole right leg, from the tip of your toe all the way up to your hip, so your toes, your calf, your thigh—contract your whole right leg. Clench it tight, hold it there, toes are curled, calf is clenched, thigh is clenched, hold it—and then release it. Again, one more time, the whole right leg: Curl the toes, clench the calf, clench the thigh, hold—and relax.

Now the left leg, whole leg, from the toe to the hip. Clench the toes, the calf, the thigh, the left leg clenches, contract and hold—and then relax and release. One more, the whole left leg. Contract and hold, and release.

Now we're going to take both legs plus your bottom, so your whole lower body. Clench your toes, tighten your calves, your thighs, clench your bottom, clenching your whole lower body, and hold it there. Feel the contraction, feel yourself pulling in and tightening, and then relax and release. One more time, contract the whole lower body, tighten it up, hold, and relax and release.

Let your lower body sink into the floor. We'll move to your abdominal muscles. Focus your awareness on your abdomen, pull your belly button towards your spine, tight to the floor, contract your abdominal muscles and hold them tight. And then release them out. One more time, belly button back to the spine, pulling your abdomen into the floor. Hold tight, and relax, release.

Move your awareness now to your right hand. Make a fist and clench your right hand tightly. Try to keep your arm relaxed, keep the forearm and the upper arm soft. Focus on the fist, the fingers, clench tightly. And then relax, and again clench the right hand, and relax. Now take the left hand, make a fist, clench it tightly. Try to keep the arm, forearm, upper arm soft, focus on the hand. Clench, and relax. One more time: Clench, and relax.

Now we'll take both hands together. Make fists, contract the hands, hold that tight, and then relax it. Again, one more time, making fists, clench your hands, and relax. Now we'll take the right hand plus the forearm so make a fist, clench your right hand and also engage the muscles of your forearm, tighten there. Feel that contraction, hold that. Then relax. Again right hand and forearm contract, and relax. Left hand and forearm—make a fist, clench the muscles of the left forearm, hold in tight, and relax. One more, left hand/ forearm contract … and release.

Now both hands and forearms. Make fists, clench the fists, clench the forearms, hold it tight there. Remember to keep breathing. And then relax. One more time, both hands, both forearms clench, and relax.

Now let's try to engage the muscles of your upper back, your upper arms, so pull your shoulder blades together, pull your arms into your side, clench your back, feel that contracting, your upper arms, your back muscles. Hold there, pressing into the floor, pressing your arms into your sides, and relax. Again, trying to isolate, keep the hands, the forearms soft, pull the upper arms into the body, the back into the floor, shoulder blades together, contract, and relax.

Bring your right shoulder up to your ear, clenching your right shoulder, contract that, and relax. One more time: Right shoulder up, contract, and release. Now the left shoulder up to your ear, contract, and release. Then pull the left shoulder up to your ear one more time, hold it there. And release. Now both shoulders, bring them up to your ears. Keep your arms relaxed, keep your back relaxed. Focus on your shoulders up to your ear; contract, release. One more time: Shoulders up to your ears, contract, remember to breathe, and release.

Now we're going to take that whole upper body—your arms, your shoulders, your back—pull your shoulders up to your ears, contract your back into the floor beneath you, clench your fists, your forearms, your upper arms squeeze into your sides, hold that—and then release. One more time, make a fist. Arms into the sides. Clench the forearms. Shoulders to the ears. Back into the floor beneath you. Clench and contract and hold that, and then relax, release. Let your upper body sink into the floor.

Let's move to the face. Squeeze your facial muscles tight. Your eyes, your mouth, clench everything in and tight and hold that, continue breathing through the nose, and now relax. One more time, the muscles of the face clench, clench your mouth tight, contract the face and hold there, remembering to breathe. And then relax.

Let's take your neck. Press the back of your head into the surface beneath you so that you're clenching the muscles of your neck. Contract there, continuing to breathe. And then relax. One more time, press the back of your head into the surface beneath you. Clench the muscles of your neck, and release.

Now let's take your whole upper body. Make fists with your hands, clench your forearms, upper arms come into your sides, shoulders up to your ears. Pull your belly button to your spine and press your back into the floor. Clench your mouth, your eyes, your neck by pressing your head back to the floor. Clench your whole upper body and hold that there tightly—contract, and then release. One more time, your whole upper body: your hands, your arms, your shoulders, your belly button, your back, your face, your neck, clench everything nice and tight and hold … and then release completely.

Now we're going to take the whole body, every muscle from the top of your head to the tips of your toes. Clench your entire body, contracting everything, remember to breathe. You're contracting your toes, your calves, your thighs, your bottom, your hands, your arms, shoulders, abdominal muscles, back, neck face—every muscle in your body. Hold it tight, and then release. One more time your whole body; contract it in and hold, and then release completely.

Feel yourself becoming heavy, sinking into the floor beneath you. Feel yourself dissolving into the floor with a sense of deep, complete relaxation. Feel the difference of having truly soft, comfortable, relaxed muscles. Take some deep breaths here and feel warm and heavy, and as if all of your muscles are soft, relaxed, open.

Take a few more deep breaths, inhaling in, and exhale away any residual stress or tension or discomfort. Inhale in a sense of being calm and relaxed and centered. And exhale away any remaining stress or tension. Feel your body become soft, sink into the floor, and just stay here, completely rested and completely relaxed for as long as you would like.

Anapana Sati (Breathing Meditation) (5 minutes)

Anapana sati, the meditation on in-and-out breathing, is a simple breathing exercise to help you focus your awareness and learn deliberate control of your thoughts. In anapana sati meditation, you use the sensation of your breath as an anchor for your focus.

Begin in a comfortable seated position. If you are comfortable sitting on the floor you can do so in a cross-legged or kneeling position. You can also sit comfortably on a chair. Key is that your posture be soft and relaxed, so that you are not distracted by discomfort. Sit with good posture, shoulders rolled down and back, chest open and soft. Palms open on your lap. Close your eyes. Focus your awareness on the physical sensation of your breath, breathing in and out through the nose. Inhale. Exhale. Focus on the sensation of air flowing through your nostrils. Inhale. Exhale. Inhale. Exhale. Inhale. Exhale. Inhale. Exhale.

If your mind wanders, if you find yourself thinking about something else, bring your awareness back to your nose, back to the way your breath feels as it flows in and out of your nostrils. Inhale. Exhale. Inhale. Exhale. Inhale. Exhale.

There's a wonderful meditation teacher named Jack Kornfield, and he says that our minds are like puppies who are not potty trained. We try to focus, and our mind runs off in a corner. We bring it back to the paper, it runs off in a corner. We bring it back to the paper, it runs off in a corner. Just continue to bring it back. Use the physical sensation of your breath to keep you grounded in this moment, this breath, this exercise. Inhale. Exhale. Keep your eyes closed, your awareness within, focusing on the sensation of your breath. Inhale. Exhale. Inhale. Exhale. Inhale. Exhale. Inhale. Exhale. Inhale. Exhale.

Use your breath as an anchor, keeping you centered in this moment. Inhale, and exhale. Slowly open your eyes. Take a few more breaths in and out. Feel a sense of being grounded in this moment, aware of how you feel right now. When you're stressed, your thoughts and fears can get away from you. A sensation-based meditation like anapana sati can bring you back to the present moment and your actual experience. You can practice it regularly to improve your ability to be centered in the moment, and you can also use it as a tool during moments of stress.

Alternate Nostril Breathing (5 minutes)

Alternate nostril breathing is a yoga breathing technique, which is great for increasing your energy level. If you're feeling tired or fatigued, or experiencing a headache or congestion, it can be a good strategy to clear your mind.

Because it crosses the midline of the body, yoga theory also holds that alternate nostril breathing helps connect the right and left brain, when you are faced with a task that requires both creative and analytical skills.

We'll begin in a comfortable seated position. If you are comfortable sitting on the floor in a cross-legged or kneeling position, you can do so. You can also sit comfortably on a chair. Key is that your posture be soft and relaxed, so that you are not distracted by discomfort. Sit with good posture, shoulders rolled down and back, chest soft and open, palms open on your lap. Bring your right hand up in front of your face, with your palm facing you. Curl in the three middle fingers of your hand, so that your thumb and pinky are extended.

Bring your thumb to your right nostril, pressing the nostril against the bridge of your nose to completely close your right nostril. Inhale in through the left nostril. Hold the breath. Release your thumb. Bring your pinky up to completely close your left nostril and exhale out. Pause, and then inhale in. Hold the breath. Release the pinky. Close the right nostril with your thumb and then exhale. Pause. Inhale. Again, switch sides. Exhale. Inhale. Switch sides. Exhale. Close your eyes. Inhale, switch sides, exhale. Pause, inhale, switch sides, pause, and exhale. Inhale, switch sides, continue moving at your own pace, switching back and forth.

You may find that one side is more congested than the other, that you breathe more clearly through one nostril. This is normal. Use your breath to work through it, to increase the clarity, to increase the airflow through each nostril. You may also find yourself a little uncomfortable, even anxious on the pause between the inhalation and the exhalation. This is normal. Breathe through it; remember that you will take another breath, that the pause is a normal part of your breathing cycle.

A couple more, and then release your hand onto your lap. Keep your eyes closed. Return to normal breathing for a few deep breaths, coming back to a sense of breathing through both nostrils. Fluid soft breathing, in and out. Then slowly open your eyes. Feel a sense of being calm but also energized, focused, awake. Set an intention to maintain this sense of calm, peaceful energy throughout the rest of your day.

Reiki Energy (Compassionate Touch) (5 minutes)

Reiki is a Japanese energy-based system, which helps you to channel the warmth and energy of your body into your own healing. We'll do a brief Reiki session to help you learn how this technique can help you to relax and work through pain or discomfort. Start in a comfortable seated position, either on a chair or on the floor, if you prefer. Bring your palms together in front of your chest, close your eyes, and take your energy within. Focus on the palms of your hands, breathing your awareness into your hands, working to feel a sense of warmth between your hands.

Take several slow breaths through your nose, breathing your awareness into your hands. Inhale. Exhale. Again inhale, and exhale. Now, slowly rub your hands together, as if you're warming them in front of a fire, getting energy from the palms of your hands. Think of a place on your body where you could use a little extra energy, a little extra focus, a little extra attention. Perhaps you've had an injury or a surgery, such as cataract surgery or a joint surgery. Perhaps you have a place of arthritis or chronic pain.

Take your hands and place them gently on the body part you'd like to focus on. Place your hands on that spot, and use your hands to focus your awareness into that part of your body. Close your eyes and take slow deliberate breaths, thinking about that part of your body; think about red blood cells rushing in with energy, white blood cells rushing in to heal, your body connecting to its capacity to heal and repair itself.

Take a nice deep inhalation. Feel yourself being connected to the health and well-being that is inside of you. Exhale completely out. Feel yourself breathing out any pain, any fear, any discomfort. Again, inhale. Exhale. As you inhale, feel yourself becoming strong, well, capable. Again, inhale … and exhale. Inhale. Exhale. Inhale. Exhale.

As you exhale, the fear, the anxiety, they wash away, out of your body, out of your mind, out of your heart. Continue breathing. Inhale. And exhale. Inhale … and exhale. Focus your awareness into that part of your body, breathing in a sense of strength and well-being, exhaling away any pain, any stress, any discomfort. Inhale. Exhale. Inhale. Exhale. One more nice deep inhale, breathing in health and well-being … exhale out completely, breathing away any residual pain. And then slowly release your hands, bringing them down onto your lap. Take one more deep breath, breathing in a sense of being strong and healthy overall. Inhale. Exhale one more time, releasing away any residual pain or fear. Now gently open your eyes.

You can do this exercise at any time and with any part of your body. If you find yourself getting caught in a loop of chronic pain, try it. It may not eliminate your pain, but it can reduce your perception and fear of it, and make it seem more manageable, helping you to feel in control of your thoughts and your body. You can also do this to support a loved one whenever you feel they may need some loving energy, and compassionate touch.

Foundational Fitness
Lecture 14

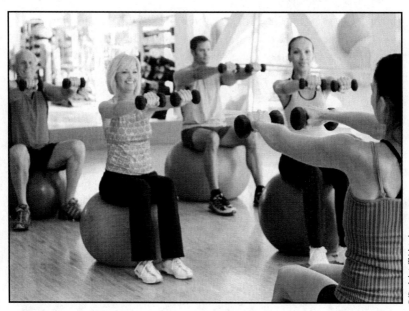

© iStockphoto/Thinkstock.

This 30-minute fitness session provides a well-balanced workout of strength training and flexibility exercises. Complete this workout 2 to 3 times per week. Add 30 minutes of gentle cardiovascular exercise, such as walking, swimming, or cycling, at least 3 days a week for a well-rounded exercise program. In this session, we use light hand weights, exercise bands, a yoga mat, an exercise ball, and a chair.

Suggested Reading

Baechle and Westcott, *Fitness Professional's Guide to Strength Training Older Adults*.

Bonura, *Pelvic Yoga*.

Foundational Fitness
Lecture 14—Transcript

Foundational Fitness (30 minutes)

This 30-minute fitness session will provide a well-balanced workout of strength-training and flexibility exercises. Complete this workout two to three times per week. Add 30 minutes of gentle cardiovascular exercise such as walking, swimming, or cycling, at least three days a week, for a well-rounded exercise routine.

We'll start with some stretching to warm up. These can all be done seated or standing, whichever you prefer. We'll do our neck first, so comfortable posture. If you're standing, feet are nice and grounded, chest is open, shoulders rolled down and back. If you're seated, comfortable posture as well, open chest, shoulders rolled down and back. We'll look to the left, over the left shoulder, opening up the side of the neck. Hold here for a couple of breaths. Feel your neck opening and stretching. Then come back to center, and let's look to the right. Breathe into that stretch. Always remember to breathe with your movements, using gentle, natural breath. And come back to center.

Let's take the left ear to the shoulder, opening up the right side of the neck. Nice long stretch. Push down to the heel with your right hand to further open up your neck. Then back to center and right ear to the shoulder, push down to the heel with the left hand. Back to center.

Now we'll do some shoulder rolls, rolling backwards. You don't need to do forward rolls—we hunch forward enough as it is over our computers and our steering wheels, so it's important to roll backward, open up the neck, open up the shoulders, get good range of motion. And then relax that. We'll do a couple shoulder shrugs, inhaling up, exhaling down, giving yourself a little massage. Inhale up, exhale down. One more up, inhale up, squeeze, and exhale down.

Now we'll do some chest and upper-body stretches; again, you can continue standing or if you're more comfortable you can sit on the chair. Fingers are interlaced, hands come behind your head, get a nice stretch here. Pull out through the elbows, opening up. And breathe into that, pulling your shoulder blades together, and then relax that, shake your arms out. Interlace your fingers behind your back, lift your chest, and look up, opening up the front of your body, creating expansiveness through the chest. Get a good stretch here. Breathe into it, really lift your chest, lift your chin, open the front of your body. And then relax, and release that. Inhale your right arm up over, stretch to the left side, the left arm stretching down the leg. The right arm lifting, if you're comfortable, look up at your middle fingertip. Create length through the right side of the body. And exhale down, take the left arm up and over, nice long stretch, look up at the left middle fingertip. Stretch down through the right hand. Breathe into it—remember to breathe, don't hold your breath. On your next exhale, release that.

We're going to take a wide-legged squat now, opening up the legs, thighs, hips. So your feet'll be nice and wide, toes are turned out. You're gonna bend down, knees about even with your ankles. You don't want to go too far down; you want to protect the knees. Hands are at the inner thighs, pressing open. Lift your chest; create openness through your body. You're stretching your inner thighs.

If you're on the chair, you're going to sit, hands at the inner thighs. Open the legs out, sit nice and tall. Either way you're getting a good stretch through the inner legs, through the hips, through the groin. Find where you feel comfortable as you're taking the squat, breathe into it for one more minute. And then inhale, come on up. We're going to take a lunge. We'll start with your left foot forward, your right foot back, you're gonna bend into the front knee and just step your legs apart as much as you feel comfortable. Knee is above the ankle; you don't wanna go forward. Protect the knee joint. Hips are squared towards the knee to center your weight, center the pelvis.

If you're seated, very similar. You've got one leg behind you, the other leg out in front, working to create some openness through the inner thighs, through the hips, again squaring your hips forward to the front knee. Working on that lunge, keeping your legs open, breathing into it, feeling your stretch through the back of the thigh.

Let's take it the other side. Right foot forward, left foot back, bending into the front knee. Back leg, the calf, the thigh, stretching. If you're seated, same thing. Right knee bent, left leg stretching behind you. And then step your feet back together, shaking your legs out.

We're going to do some light resistance training, using hand weights. Your weights should be between 2 and 5pounds to start; gradually you can increase that to between 5 and 20 pounds, depending on your ability. We'll start here with one set of 8 repetitions. You can work up to 12. When that feels comfortable, you'll work up to three sets of 8 to 12 repetitions. First, as it's comfortable, one set of 8 repetitions, then two sets of 8 repetitions, then three sets of 8 repetitions, working up to 12. Then begin to add more weight, as you feel stronger, as it feels more comfortable.

You've got light hand weights, just comfortable ones, we're going to start with a squat. A weight is in each hand. The weights should be the same, you want to make sure they're evenly weighted for each hand so that your body is balanced. Your feet are a little bit wider than hip-width apart. If you'd like, you've got the chair here for balance, if you need to just do one hand at a time, if you're worried about your balance and your stability.

Your feet are a little bit wider than hip-width apart. Solid stance, toes forward, arms by your sides, fingers curled gently around the weights. Your wrists are neutral, not bent. You want to make sure and protect your wrists. Pull your belly button into your spine to stabilize your core, give you good strong, solid balance. Slowly, with control, we're going to bend at the knees; keep your chest open and your torso lifted. Don't allow your upper body to sink forward, don't allow your knees to bend too far forward, feel what's comfortable. You're coming down as if you are sitting in a chair. Then you come back up slowly and with control. We're going to do seven more. Take the squat, and come back up. Down for three, and up. Down for four, and up. Five, up. Six, up. Seven, up. And eight, and back up. If it feels like, that's OK. You can always use a heavier hand weight, but it's also good to start small. Build your strength up. Let's prevent injury by moving slowly, being gentle, giving your body time to increase your strength and your ability level.

We're going to do heel raises now so your feet are a little closer together, directly under your hips. Again, the chair is here beside you if you want to do one weight center in front of you and use the chair for support. Listen to your body, you balance needs. Weights are by your sides, wrists are neutral, belly button into the spine to stabilize your torso, create control of your core. With control, you're going to lift up onto your toes and then lower your heels back to your floor. Again, if you need some support, holding the chair as you lift, and go down. That's two; let's do six more. Lift, and down. Lift for four, and down. Lift for five, and down. Lift for six, down. Seven, down. One more, lift up for eight, and down.

We're going to use some exercise bands for a few moments. These are great for resistance training. Because they come in different levels of strength, so you'll look to see is it a light, is it a medium, is it a heavy. Start with a lower level resistance band and work up to increased resistance. They come in an open strip but you can tie them to form a loop for other exercises. We'll be using our first exercise with a loop. They can provide a challenging workout, but they also offer a workout, you can carry them in your suitcase, you can have them in your desk at work, and there's a really low risk of injury—you can't drop them on your foot, or hurt yourself lifting too heavy a weight.

These are great for the hips in particular. You can do some really great exercises for the hips, and we're going to start doing hip abduction using the resistance bands. You can do it either seated or standing. I'll show you both. If you're going to do it standing, you will also be challenging your balance to further train your core-body muscles.

Again, we've got it tied in a circle. It needs to be sufficient to let you get into the band to let you have it around your ankles with your feet about hip-width apart, but be small enough that you've actually got some resistance then when you move. If you're seated, good posture, feet firmly planted about hip-width apart. We're gonna put it around our ankles, feet are nice and firm. We're going to plant the left foot. If you're standing and you want the chair for support, you've got it there to help you. You're going to have your hand at the waist. We're going to stretch the right leg to the side, pressing against the band, hold it for a few breaths and then release it back. If you need to drop your toe for a moment, that's OK, find your balance. Lift it out to the side, relax it down.

If you're seated, what that looks like is that you've got your feet there. Left foot grounded, pull out with the right leg. Relax, one more, whether you're standing or seated, out to the side, and relax. Let's do the opposite side now. Again, plant your right foot whether you're standing or seated, plant it firmly. Lift your left leg out to the side, press against the band. Hold it there for a few breaths, and release. Hold it there for a few breaths as you lift it up, release it down. Two more. Lift it out to the side, and release. One more time, lift it out to the side, and release it down.

We're going to do hip adduction now, moving the opposite way. Firmly plant your left foot, and you're going to take your right leg across the midline, pressing against the band. Again, you've got the chair here for balance. Use it the first few times to make sure you feel stable. Start with your right leg in front, and then cross across, challenging that inner thigh. Hold that there, and release. If you're comfortable with your balance, hands at your hip, take that across, and release.

If you're seated, what that looks like is the left foot's planted, right foot's in front, you're going to have to lift a little higher so that you can take it across the knee, and release, whether standing or sitting, one more time, take it across. And release. Let's do the opposite side. Again, chair for balance for the first time that you try to make sure you feel stable. Take the left foot in front of the right; cross the midline. Feel yourself working the inner thigh, and release. Take number two if your balance is good, hands at the waist, and release. Two more, press across the midline, and release. One more time, press across the midline, and release. Go ahead and take the band off of your legs; we'll do some upper-body work.

We'll start with bicep curls. You've got the weights in your hands, and we're going to do these first with the hand weights, and then we're going to try these with resistance bands, so that you can see the different options available to you for doing biceps curls.

With weights, stand firmly with your feet about hip width apart, nice solid stance. You can also do this seated on a chair if you feel more comfortable. Upper-body movement is the same either way. Hold one weight in each hand, with your palms facing forward. Keep your elbows into your sides, press them into your ribcage for stability, and then slowly with control curl the weights up to your shoulders. Slowly release down to your sides. Curl up, and release down. Curl up, release down. Curl up for five, release down. Up for six, release down. Up for seven, release down. One more, up for eight, and release down.

Now, we're going to try doing the curl with the resistance band and I'm going to demonstrate this one seated so you can see but you can also do it standing. You're going to have your band under your feet, nice and firm, one hand on each side of the band. You're going to have your arms solid beside you, your posture should be good, nice and lifted and press the feet down solidly. Slowly with control lift your palms up. And then curl down. Again, keep your elbows into your sides to support your upper body to keep your arms controlled. Curl up, and down. Curl up, and down. Curl up, and down. Curl up, and down. Two more. Curl up, and down. Curl up, and down. Very nice.

Alright we're going to do a shoulder press, another upper-body exercise. Again, seated or standing, either is fine. You're going to hold a dumbbell in each hand. You're standing, your feet are about hip-width apart, firmly planted into the floor for solid posture. If you're seated, good solid posture on the chair. Bring your arms out to the sides in goal post position, so elbow to shoulder, nice straight line, controlled bend at the elbow so that it's an even 90-degree angle, wrists are neutral and straight, protect your wrists, you don't want them to be folded forward or back. Nice straight posture. Belly button into your spine to stabilize your core. Slowly, with control, lift your arms over your head. Then bring them back to goalpost. Lift, and back to goalpost. Lift, and back to goalpost. That's three.

If you're seated it's the same way. Nice solid posture, and you lift, and goalpost. That's four. Lift, goalpost, that's five. Lift, goalpost, that's six. Lift, back to goalpost, that's seven. Lift, back to goalpost. That's eight.

Now we'll do triceps kick-back, and we'll do each arm one at a time. You're next to your chair and you're going to place the right knee on the chair, bend at the waist and place your right hand on the chair for balance. Keep your left a little bit bent so that knee doesn't lock and it's comfortable. The weight's in your left hand with your left elbow close to your side, again wrist is neutral. Again, wrist is neutral. I know I keep saying that but it's very easy to accidentally turn the wrist out or turn it in. You want to keep it neutral and keep it comfortable to protect the wrist. Keeping the elbow in place at your hip, extend your forearm back until it is almost straight. Don't lock your elbow. Keep your elbow at your hip, and then lower the arm back to standing position. Again lift and then bring it back, that's two. Lift, bring it back, that's three. You're looking down at the floor, neutral neck, comfortable spine. Lift, bring it back that's four. Lift, bring it back, that's five. Lift, bring it back, that's six. Lift, bring it back, that's seven. Lift, bring it back, that's eight.

If you're prefer to stay seated for the triceps kick-back you can bend forward a little bit, bend forward a little bit, put one elbow on your knee, the right elbow is going to be in at the hip at the waist, and you're going to bend your body forward a little bit. Take it back. Elbow stays in and release. Two, release. Three, release. Four, again your neck is neutral, your spine is neutral. Release. Five, keeping control of the elbow and wrist, release. Six, release. Seven, release. Eight, release. Very good.

Now let's switch sides. Place your left knee on the chair, then bend at the waist, and place your left hand on the chair for balance. Keep your right leg slightly bent. Hold the weight in your right hand. Place your right elbow close to your side, wrist is neutral.

Keeping your elbow in place at your hip, extend your forearm backward until it is almost straight. Be careful not to lock your elbow. Keep your elbow at your hip, while you lower your arm to the starting position.

Core body strength is an important part of any fitness program, to support your posture through strengthening the muscles of your abdomen and your back. We'll start with abdominal exercises on an exercise ball. Look for a ball that allows you to sit comfortably without too much bend at the knee.

They generally come in three heights, so look for the height that's right for you.

We're going to do pelvic tilts forward and back. Center yourself on the ball, legs spread wide, open, relaxed posture, chest open, shoulders rolled down and back, and we'll roll the pelvis forward, tucking the belly button into the spine, and then roll the pelvis backward, stretching the front of the body. Tuck in, roll back. Tuck in, roll back. Tuck in, feeling yourself lengthening the lower part of your back, and then roll back, creating length and openness in the front of your body. One more time, tuck in, and roll back.

Come back to sitting with your legs wide, chest lifted, strong open posture, and engage the muscles of your core and legs to gently bounce. Staying upright while bouncing challenges the small muscles of the back; feel how it also engages your glutes and thighs. If you use a ball as a desk chair, you will be challenging your core muscles to stay upright throughout the day. You can also add in a few bounces each hour to increase the challenge.

Now we'll do a backbend over the ball. This is a great, supported backbend, which allows you to really open up the front of the body for an expansive stretch; you may want to do this near a chair or wall so that you have something to grab if you feel yourself start to roll, or need help coming back up

Come forward to the front of the ball, and make sure your feet are firmly planted, about hip-width apart, for a solid stance. You should be on a solid, non-slippery surface, so that the ball doesn't roll under you. Slowly roll the ball forward under your body as you lean backward and come back to gently relaxing over the ball. If you're feeling comfortable you can take your arms up over your head and really sink into the stretch; get a nice, long stretch, sinking into the ball, feeling the front of your body open up. Just relax here for a couple of breaths, allowing yourself to breathe naturally and gently.

When you're ready to come up, bring your hands up to your hips, bring your belly button back to your spine to engage your core, stabilize your back, tuck your chin in and very slowly roll up, rolling the ball back under you to come back up to sitting. Remember to be gentle with your abdominal muscles and your back.

We'll come to the floor now and we'll start with one more arm exercise: seated rows on the floor using resistance bands. You'll have the band and you're on the floor on your mat, feet a little bit wider than your hips. The band is untied this time. Stretch it around the soles of your feet and then cross the resistance bands so that you take the incoming around your left foot in your right hand, and the incoming around your right foot in your left hand. Your arms are stretched out in front of you over your legs. Bend your elbows slowly while pulling towards your hips, and then slowly release. Bend and pull, slowly release. If you're not comfortable being on the floor, you can wrap around a doorknob while seated on a chair in front of the door and pull the band toward you in the same way.

Let's take five more. Pull, release, keep your elbows in, your posture nice and tall. Four, and release. Five, release. Six, and release. Seven, and release. And eight, and release. Very nice. Now we'll do some additional core-body work on the floor.

We'll start with a plank position. You'll be on your hands and knees, hands about shoulder-width apart, knees about shoulder-width apart, and your fingers are spread wide, palms pressed into the ground below you as if they're suction cups, really planted firmly. That takes some of the weight off the wrists and protects the wrists. You can stay here if this feels comfortable, just staying in a tabletop position, keeping the knees on the ground for extra support. If you'd like to further challenge your core, you're going to step your feet back onto your toes, and press back through your heels. Your weight is centered, shoulders directly above the wrists, pulling the belly button towards the spine for stability. We'll just stay here for about five deep breaths, feel the strength of the core body. Belly button towards the spine. Breathe into that. Don't hold your breath; breathe naturally and gently through the nose, pulling back through the heels. Then bring the knees down and we'll take one more plank on your elbows this time. You're going to bring your hands down, elbows and wrists down, nice flat upper arms, again pressing the fingers nice and strong. You can stay on the knees if this feels challenging. If you'd like to take it further, again stretch back through the legs, pulling through the heels. Five deep breaths here pulling the belly button towards the spine for stability. Remember to breathe, don't hold your breath. Then we'll come down and we're going to come onto our backs.

Your feet are about hip-width apart, planting firmly into the ground. Knees are bent gently, and you can place your hands beside you for some support as you gently roll back, use your elbows if you'd like to gently bring yourself back onto the floor, flat back. Hands are beside you, palms facing down, fingers spread wide, feet hip-width apart. Keep your gaze directly up, your neck neutral. Never turn your head while you're in bridge pose. Plant the hands and feet and gently lift your bottom up towards the ceiling, pulling the belly button towards your spine to stabilize the core, you're lifting the glutes. Then we'll come down. If you'd like you can change the angle by bringing your feet in a little bit, find what feels comfortable as an angle for you. We'll lift up, pushing up nice and high. Belly button towards the spine, stable core, hands pressing towards the ground, your gaze is directly up to protect the neck. And relax down. Let's just do one more, lift up nice and high. Breathe into it; remember to breathe. And relax down.

Now we'll talk what's called thread the needle. This is a great opener for the low back, the hips. Keep your left foot planted, cross your right ankle over your left knee. Just let the right knee open out to the side. This might be enough of a stretch for you. If it is, stay here. If you're feeling comfortable, you want to challenge yourself a little bit more, you're going to bring the left knee towards you, bring your hands through the legs to wrap around your left thigh. This might be where you stay. If you'd like a little bit more challenge, bring your head up towards your feet. You'll feel this through the hips, the thighs, the low back. You have sciatic nerve pain, this is a really great stretch to do, to open up that area. And then release the head down, release the left foot down, release the right foot and we'll change sides. Right foot solid, cross the left ankle over, you might stay here if this feels like a good stretch for you. If you want to take it further you'll lift the knee towards you. Bring the arms through and around the right thigh. And then again if you want a little bit more of a stretch lift the head up. Breathe here a couple of deep breaths. And then relax your head down, release the arms, bring the right foot down, left foot down. We're going to come up to sitting. Bring your hands onto your thighs very gently, tuck your chin, and roll up if you'd like abdominal work. If that doesn't feel good, the other option is to roll onto one side, press up through the hand to protect the low back. Always listen to your body. Find what feels comfortable for you.

We're going to do some pelvic floor exercises now to strengthen your pelvic floor and prevent or help overcome incontinence. If you're on the floor, comfortable, cross-legged position, you can also sit on a chair if that feels more comfortable. Focus your awareness at your pelvic floor. Remember you're isolating the muscles of your pelvic floor as if you're trying to suppress the flow of gas. You're going to come to the pelvic floor, keep the thighs, the bottom, the stomach soft and we're going to lift up and hold for 5, 4, 3, 2, 1 and release. Again, contract and hold for n, this is a really great stretch to do, to open up that area. And then release the head down, release the left foot down, release the right foot and we'll change sides. Right foot solid, cross the left ankle over, you might stay here if this feels like a good stretch for you. If you want to take it further you'll lift the knee towards you. Bring the arms through and around the right thigh. And then again if you want a little bit more of a stretch lift the head up. Breathe here a couple of deep breaths. And then relax your head down, release the arms, bring the right foot down, left foot down. We're going to come up to sitting. Bring your hands onto your thighs very gently, tuck your chin, and roll up if you'd like abdominal work. If that doesn't feel good, the other option is to roll onto one side, press up through the hand to protect the low back. Always listen to your body. Find what feels comfortable for you.

We're going to do some pelvic floor exercises now to strengthen your pelvic floor and prevent or help overcome incontinence. If you're on the floor, comfortable, cross-legged position, you can also sit on a chair if that feels more comfortable. Focus your awareness at your pelvic floor. Remember you're isolating the muscles of your pelvic floor as if you're trying to suppress the flow of gas. You're going to come to the pelvic floor, keep the thighs, the bottom, the stomach soft and we're going to lift up and hold for 5, 4, 3, 2, 1 and release. Again, contract and hold for 5, 4, 3, 2, 1, release. Again, contract and hold for 5,4, 3, 2, 1 release. One more, lift and hold for 5, 4, 3, 2, 1, release.

Now we're going to try what's a quick flick, a flash contraction. You're going to get your awareness at your pelvic floor, and we're going to contract-release, contract-release, contract-release, contract-release, contract-release. Now we're going to do one long hold. This helps build endurance of the pelvic floor muscles. Lift up and hold now for 10, 9, 8, 7, 6, remember to breathe, 5, 4, 3, 2, 1 and release.

We'll finish our exercise routine now with a few gentle stretches to relax your body, work the range of motion in your joints, and quiet your mind. You can remain seated on the floor or sit comfortable on a chair. Gentle twist to start, bring your left hand to your right knee, right hand behind you either to the floor or to the side of the chair, and just gently twist to look towards the right shoulder. The movement comes through the torso, neck is very gentle and relaxed. And back to center, let's twist the other direction. And back to center.

Stretch your legs out in front of you. If you're on the chair, legs are comfortable in front of you. We're going to roll the ankles and the wrists in. And then roll them out just getting mobility in the joints. Then we're going to stretch the fingers and the toes, open wide and curl them all in. Stretch them nice and wide, and then just come back to a comfortable seated position. Palms open on your lap, close your eyes, we'll take a few deep breaths to quiet your mind. Take a nice deep inhalation into the lower lobes of your lungs, soft abdomen, and then exhale away any stress or residual tension. Inhale in a nice deep breath, feel yourself calm, centered, exhale away any stress, any frustration. One more deep breath, inhale in a sense of being centered, a sense of accomplishment for taking care of your health and becoming more fit, more healthy. Exhale out.

We've done a balanced workout to stretch and tone your legs, arms, core body, and pelvic floor. Feel a sense of accomplishment for the work that you've done today. Complete this workout two to three times per week and remember to add 30 minutes of gentle cardiovascular exercise, such as walking, swimming, or cycling at least three times a week for a well-rounded exercise routine. Great job!

Core Strength and Balance
Lecture 15

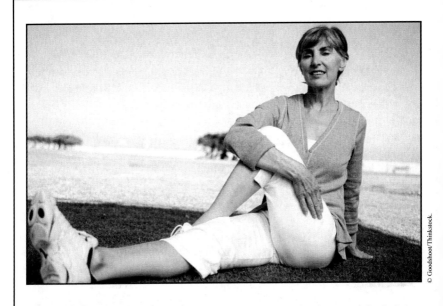

© Goodshoot/Thinkstock.

Maintaining core strength and balance is fundamental in helping you maintain independence. In this lecture, we will focus on physical exercises that improve your posture and strengthen the muscles of the core and back to improve overall balance. The lecture includes two 15-minute sessions, one chair based and one floor based. The chair-based session is gentle and accessible for everyone, regardless of flexibility or current fitness level. The floor-based routine uses yoga and Pilates exercises to support you in further developing core strength and balance.

Suggested Reading

Austin, *Pilates for Every Body*.

Schatz, *Back Care Basics*.

Core Strength and Balance
Lecture 15—Transcript

Chair Routine (10 minutes)

Maintaining core strength and balance is fundamental in helping you maintain independence. In this session, we will focus on physical exercises to improve your posture and strengthen the muscles of the core and back, to improve overall balance. This chair-based core strength and balance session is gentle and accessible for everyone, regardless of your flexibility or current fitness level.

We'll start seated on a chair in a simple sitting position. Knees are above the ankles, chest is open, shoulders are rolled down, hands are going to be on your stomach because we'll start with abdominal breathing. Abdominal breathing is key in building core strength. Take a nice deep inhalation, breathing into the lower lobes of your lungs, and as your inhale let your stomach actually soften and expand, giving the lungs space to fill into the lower parts of the body.

As you exhale, belly button back to the spine, and pushing the air out of your body. Inhale, breathe deeply. Exhale, belly button back to the spine. Inhale. And exhale. Inhale again, and exhale. We're breathing in and out through the nose, slow, deliberate controlled breathing.

Now we'll take a staff pose, so your knees are above your ankles, feet are pressing into the floor, roll your shoulders down and back and actually bring your hands to the sides of the chair and hold onto the sides of the chair, using that as an anchor to further roll your shoulders back. Bring your belly button back to the spine, tuck your chin in. And feel solid through your core, centered, grounded, the belly button back to the spine to really engage the muscles of the abdomen. Feel tall here, lengthening the back of the neck. The chin is pressing into the throat. Throat lock is though in yoga theory to engage the thyroid. Take one more breath here, and then relax, come back up to center.

We're going to take a couple of twists to open up the torso. Give some rotation to the internal muscles, the internal organs. Left hand at the outside of the right knee, right hand behind you, twist and rotate; you're rotating through the torso, through the chest. The head and neck follow gently. Neck is comfortable and relaxed. Breathe into it here. Couple more deep breaths, in and out through the nose. And then back to center, and let's take the other side. Rotating to look over the left shoulder, rotating through the torso, neck and head follow gently. Breathe into it. And come back to center.

Bring your hands to your hips. We're going to do a couple of leg lifts because these help to strengthen the upper thighs, the hips, engaging the lower muscles in the abdomen to help strengthen your lower body which will help with your balance and your core stability. Ground your left foot into the floor and lift your right leg, strengthen the knee, and then lift up off of the chair. Try to lift the thigh off of the chair so you're really engaging. Breathe into that; try to remember to breathe, don't contract your breath. Relax the leg. Press the right foot into the ground, lift and straighten the left leg, and then lift the left leg off the chair. Breathe into that. And relax the left leg. Take the right leg again, straighten, lift, lift off the chair. And release. Left side again, point your toe, lift up. Remember to keep breathing. This is another simple exercise that you can do at your desk that you can do while you're working, or when you're at home relaxing, watching television. Great way to get small movements into your day. Release, one more set. Lift the right leg, lift off the chair, really engage the muscles of your legs, your hips. Relax it. Last one, left leg, lift up off the chair. And relax it down.

Let's take a seated bicycle. You're going to interlace your fingers. Bring your hands behind your head. We're going to be working the hips again, also working the whole core. You're going to lift your left knee, bring your right elbow towards your knee. Then come back to center. We're going to move this with our breath now. We're going to exhale as we lift and inhale as we open back up. Exhale, contract, breath out of your body so you can contract through the core, inhale open back up. Exhale contract, inhale open back up. Couple more. Exhale, contract; inhale open. Exhale contract; inhale open. Exhale contract; inhale open. Last one. Exhale contract; inhale open.

Hands stay behind your head, elbows are out, sit up nice and straight, chest is open, belly button back to the spine. Let's stretch to the left as you exhale. Inhale up to center. Exhale to the right. Inhale up to center. Keep your posture open, your belly button back to the spine, nice tall open posture. Exhale left, inhale center. Exhale right, inhale center. Couple more. Exhale left, inhale center. Exhale right, inhale center. Relax your arms, shake them out. Let's take the arms straight out to the sides, and you're going to pull your shoulder blades together, bringing together the muscles in your back, strengthening the middle of your back. We're going to hold this for a couple of breaths. Keep your neck open and relaxed. Keep your shoulders down, shoulder blades pulled together, isolating the center of your back. Relax. Pull together again, bringing the shoulder blades together. And relax. Again, shoulder blades together, and relax. One more, pull the shoulder blades together, and relax, relax your arms down. Shake them out. Get rid of any stress of tension in the arms.

Now we're going to bring the arms up to goalpost. Elbows are bent, fingers are spread wide. Open up, pulling the elbows back, pull your shoulders rolled down and back to pull the shoulder blades together. You're opening the chest; you're strengthening the back. Hold this here for several deep breaths, breathing in and out through the nose. Keep the belly button back toward the spine so you're engaging the core. Breathe into it. And then relax the arms, shake them out.

Now come forward a little bit on your chair. Feet are a little bit wider, hands are on your knees. We're going to do stomach pump. You may remember this from one of our lectures. You're going to take a nice deep inhalation, let the stomach soften and relax. Exhale all the way out, belly button back to the spine, push the air out of your body. Once the air is out you're going to contract your abdominal muscles back and forth. Inhale breathe, exhale belly button back to the spine and pump. Be careful of your breath; if you need to breathe more regularly just pause, inhale. Exhale back to the spine. Take it again. If you have hypertension, a history of panic attacks, be aware of your breath; breathe as you need to. Inhale. Exhale back to the spine. Pump again. This is a great exercise for toning the muscles of the abdomen. Great thing to build into your day. One more, inhale, exhale, belly button back to the spine. Then pump your stomach; contract, use the muscles of your core. And relax.

Come back to a comfortable position. Palms open on your lap. Shoulders rolled down and back. Chest is open. Close your eyes. Let's take a couple of deep, soft breaths here, inhaling in, letting your stomach expand, let your breath fill your body, exhaling out. Inhale; exhale. One more. Inhale, and exhale all the way out. Soft, gentle breathing. Feel a sense of strength through the core of your body, helping you to feel strong and empowered. You can work on your balance and core strength throughout the day simply by practicing abdominal breathing and being diligent about good posture. One more nice deep breath. And then exhale all the way out and relax.

Core Strength and Balance Floor Routine (20 minutes)

Maintaining core strength and balance is key to supporting the ability to maintain independence. In this session, we will focus on physical exercises that improve the posture, strengthen the muscles of the core and the back, and improve overall balance. This floor-based routine uses yoga and Pilates exercises to support you in further developing your core strength and balance.

We'll start on the floor, on a hands-and-knees position. Come onto your mat, knees directly under your hips. Bend at the waist, hands directly under your shoulders. Nice flat back, neck is neutral, looking down beneath you. Just take a tabletop position here. Feeling the stability of your back muscles, pull your belly button up towards your spine to strengthen and engage the muscles of your core.

We'll do a gentle stretch first with cat cow pose. First, you'll drop the belly down, lift the chest and chin and look up. Then as you exhale, as if you're an angry cat, roll the spine, arching the back, tuck the chin in. Inhale, drop the back down, lift the chest and chin. Exhale, roll the spine, tuck the chin in. Inhale, drop the belly, lift the chest and chin. Exhale, roll the spine, tuck the chin in. And come back to a solid tabletop position.

We're going to take some balances here, engaging the muscles of the core. Belly button to the spine, lift your left leg, straight out behind you at hip height. Then if you feel solid, right arm out in front, straight out of the shoulder, focus your gaze at your right middle fingertip. Working on stability here, breathe into that. Don't hold your breath, remember to breathe fluidly, naturally. And then exhale down. Let's take the other side, right leg out behind you. Left arm out in front. Focus your gaze at your left middle fingertip. And release the hand, release the knee. Let's take the other side again. Left leg out, right arm out, focus your gaze at your middle fingertip. Stretching from toe to fingertip. Using your core to stay stable and solid. Release down. Other side. Point through the right toe and the left fingertip. And release the hand. Release the foot.

We're going to take a plank position. Hands will be directly under your shoulders, fingers spread nice and wide, palms pressing to the mat beneath you to be solid and to protect the wrists by spreading the weight throughout the hands. Knees are hip width apart, toes are curled under, and you'll lift the knees, press back through the heels, your weight is grounded over the hands, centered at the core of your body, belly button pulling towards the spine for stability. Breathe here, five deep breaths. Then bring your knees down.

We're going to take a side plank, first with knee support. You're going to bring your left knee to center, your left hand in front of the knee, and turn your right foot out, toes are facing forward, back heel is aligned with the toes of your left foot. Then you're going to lift the right arm up. If you're comfortable, look up at your middle fingertip, opening up through the shoulder. Make sure you're got nice alignment from the shoulder to the elbow to the wrist. Opening up the front of your body. Then release that hand down. We'll take it on the other side, so you've got your right hand solid, right knee down, left foot it back, toe pointing out. If you're comfortable left arms opens up, looking up at the left middle fingertip. Couple breaths here, remember to breathe. Never hold your breath. And then release that hand down.

Now we're going to take a side plank. You can keep using the knees for support if that feels more comfortable. If you'd like to try some additional challenge, come into your plank. Bring your right hand to center. Rotate onto the side of your right foot; lift your left arm up. Feet are stacked, gaze is centered and neutral, lifting up through the left fingertips, hold here. Feel nice and strong and stable, keeping your hip lifted, don't let it sink. Lift up to stay solid. And then bring the hands back to plank, and we'll take the other side, so you're centering your hands again in a solid plank. Left hand comes to center, rolling onto the edge of the left foot, lift the right arm. Nice, solid posture. Again, perfectly fine to do this with knee support a second time. Go where you feel comfortable. And then back to plank, bring your knees and come flat down onto the mat.

We're going to take a couple of core exercises here, opening up the front of the body, strengthening the muscles of the back. Feet are about hip-width apart. Toes are pointed. Gently lift your chest up. Open the front of your body. Couple deep breaths here. Keep your gaze forward; you're pulling your shoulder blades together; elbows stay into your ribs. Relax down for a second, let yourself rest on one cheek for a moment. Then back to center. Push up a little bit higher. Lift your chest and chin. Cobra pose here, elbows stay in, opening the front of your body. And exhale down. This time you're going to lift your hands off the mat, let them hover. Inhale, lift your chest and chin, pulling your shoulder blades together, pulling your chest forward. You'll feel this engage through the middle of your back in particular. Exhale down, rest on one side of your face again for a moment. Then back to center, stretch your arms out in front of you, point your toes. If this feels uncomfortable, go back to doing just the upper body, but if you'd like the additional challenge on your inhale lift your toes, lift your arms, pulling together through the middle of the back, through your glutes, lifting up. Breathe into it. And exhale down. Bring your hands beside you. You're going to lift and press back into a child's pose, resting your hips on your heels, let your head relax down between your arms. Let your back soften. Breathe into it. Child's pose is a great pose for lower back discomfort.

Now we'll come to a downward facing dog. You're going to come up into a tabletop position, knees under your hips, hands directly under your shoulders. Fingers are spread very wide, pressing through the center of your palms, curl your toes under, lift your knees, press your weight back towards your hips. Relax your head down between your arms. Your heels are probably not touching the floor; if they're touching the floor your legs are probably too close and you should step your feet back a little bit. You want to feel a stretch down the backs of the legs, down the calves. You're pushing your weight back towards your hips to lengthen the spine from the base of the spine to the base of the neck, so you're not over your hands, you're pressing back, creating length. Breathe into it, a couple of deep breaths here. Feel yourself becoming longer, almost taller in your spine, creating openness. Then bring your knees back down and rest one more time in child's pose. Letting your body sink into the floor, letting yourself rest and relax for a moment, and then gently come up and we're going to come onto our backs.

Your feet are about hip-width apart, knees are bent, very gently you're going to roll down onto your back. Hands are flat beside you on each side, palms facing down. We'll start with a bridge pose. You're going to be looking up at the ceiling. Never turn your head in bridge pose. Knees are bent comfortably; feet are planted firmly on the floor, feet are hip-width apart, hands are beside you. Press your hands and feet and lift your bottom up, engaging the muscles of the glutes, the backs of the legs, engaging the muscles of your abdomen, strengthening the back, pulling the belly button into the spine, really feeling your core contracting, engaged. Breathe here for five deep breaths, in and out through the nose. Then exhale one vertebra at a time, slowly lowering back down to the mat. Then again, pressing your hands and feet, lift your bottom up one more time. If you're comfortable you can actually walk your shoulders under a little bit to lift up higher, further challenging your low back, your glutes to lift and engage. Breathe into it. And then release the arms back out. One vertebra at a time, walk your spine back down, and release all the way, stretch your legs out.

Bring your left knee into your chest, arms wrapped around the knee. Nice, long stretch here, great for the low back. If you have any issues with sciatic nerve pain this is a great exercise to do. It's also called wind-relieving post, so it's normal if you experience any release of wind in this pose. Great for your digestive system. And then release that, let's take the other leg, bring the knee in, wrap your arms around the leg. This is another stretch that you can modify if you're at work, sitting in your chair, you could bring one knee up to your chest. Great way to get a low back stretch during the middle of your workday. Then bring both knees, wrap your arms around your legs, hug your knees to your chest. If you're feeling comfortable, you want to press, to push a little farther, you can tuck your chin in, lift your head up. But be mindful of your neck. If you have any neck issues, be very very gentle.

Keep the head centered on the ground. Bring the head back down. We're going to open the arms out to the sides, and we're going to take the knees over to the right, and let them hover just a couple of inches off the ground, engaging your abdominal muscles, the obliques in particular, great for toning the waistline in particular. Breathe here; try to keep your left shoulder on the mat. Keep your torso and your gaze square and centered. Come back to center; let's go the other direction. Hovering. Keep your right shoulder down; keep your gaze and your torso centered. Back to center, let's do one or two more on each side. Dropping over to the right. Back to center. And then dropping over to the left, moving with control, moving slowly, being mindful and respectful of your body. Back to center. One more on each side. Moving over to the right, let it hover. If you'd like additional challenge, you can straighten your legs out. Notice how you'll have to push harder through your right arm to maintain that. Bend the knees to bring them back to center. Drop over to the left. Once you hover if you'd like the additional challenge, straighten the legs out, pushing through the left arm to give you balance to keep you stable. Bend the knees; bring them back to center.

Now arms nice and open and wide, and this time we're going to drop the knees all the way over to the right; let them completely soften and relax. And then drop your gaze over to the left arm, so that you've got a nice rotation through the torso, opening the body up to relax and rest. Breathe into that. Just take several deep breaths here. This is a great stretch to do at night before bed. Just lying in your bed, drop your hips to one side, look to the other. Close your eyes and just sink into it. Let your body absorb that deep relaxing. Back to center, moving gently, let's drop the knees over to the left, gaze is to the right. Just relax into it; sink and absorb. Then come back to center.

Bring your knees to your chest and we're going to take something called the happy baby pose. You're going to lift your feet up, and then bring your knees towards your armpits, bring your hands to the insides of your feet, and pull your knees down towards your armpits. You're like a little happy baby in a crib, opening up your hips. This pose can actually make you feel very vulnerable because you're opening up through the core, so if you find any emotionality coming up, that's OK. Just breathe into it. Let yourself feel your hips opening up, feel your body relaxing and sinking into it, and just go into your breath. Relax into your breath. Then you're going to bring your knees together in front of your chest, arms wrapped around the knees. If you've got any issues and you're uncomfortable about coming up, you're just going to gently roll over to the side and press yourself up.

But if you're comfortable, you feel confident in your back and neck and you want to try one more exercise here, you're actually going to rock and roll. Give yourself a massage of your spine. Great way to really work all the muscles of your back. Take a couple of rocks and rolls, and then come on up and pause, knees are bent, toes are pointed; you've got your chest lifted, nice tall spine, lifting up, engaging through the core, belly button to the spine. This is boat pose; if you're solid here and you want to challenge it, stretch out through the arms, stretching through the fingertips. If you really want to push, straighten out through the legs. Keep lifting through the belly button and the chest to keep your posture strong and solid and stable. Then knees into the chest.

We're going to take a low squat. Feet are nice and wide. Toes are turned out; hands are inside your knees. Palms pressed together. Lifting through the chest. You can have your bottom down, but if you can lift up that's great; if you can have your heels on the ground, wonderful, great way to really stretch here. Couple more deep breaths; feel yourself opening up your hips. Then relax your bottom down. Come back to a cross-legged position on the floor, palms open in your lap, chest lifted, and take a couple of deep breaths. Just close your eyes. Feel a sense of being stable, centered, strong, your chest is open; shoulders are rolled down and back. Feel the openness of your posture, the strength of your core. Take one more nice, deep inhalation. And exhale completely out. And set an intention to feel strong and balanced throughout the rest of your day.

Workplace Fitness
Lecture 16

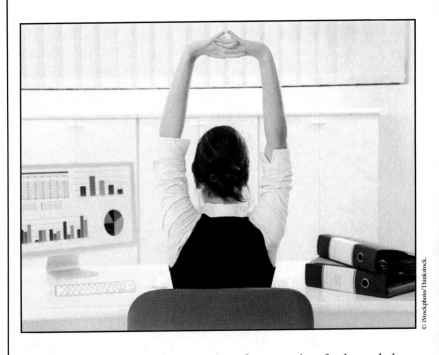

© iStockphoto/Thinkstock.

This lecture includes three 10-minute fitness sessions for the workplace, one each for standing up and moving, managing stress, and getting energized. If possible, take a walk around the block or your office building to add some cardiovascular exercise.

Suggested Reading

Archer and Gonzales, *Fitness 9 to 5*.

Kneale, *Desk Pilates*.

Zeer and Montagna, *Office Spa*.

Workplace Fitness
Lecture 16—Transcript

Stand Up and Move (10 minutes)

You have a busy day ahead of you. You want to do a workout, but you aren't sure where or how you will find the time. If you don't have time for anything else, try this 10-minute workout to stretch and tone. Add two quick 10-minute walks at lunchtime and dinnertime, and you'll have achieved 30 minutes of exercise in minimal time. You've done a great job in making health a priority, however busy your schedule.

Let's do a few stretches to open up and get started. If you prefer to stay seated, you're in a comfortable position on a chair, chest open, shoulders rolled down and back, nice open posture. If you feel comfortable, we'll do these exercises standing, so you'll be in standing position, feet a little bit wider than hip width, firmly planted into the floor. Either way, posture's open and relaxed, shoulders rolled down and back, chest open. We'll start with some neck stretches. Look to the right, opening up your neck. Breathe here, close your eyes if you feel comfortable to just relax into that. Then look to the left, opening up the other side of the neck, relaxing gently into that stretch.

Then come back to center and we'll take shoulder shrugs a couple of times to open up the shoulders. Inhale, squeeze up. Exhale down. Inhale up, exhale down. Inhale up, exhale down. Inhale up, exhale down. One more. Inhale, squeeze up, and exhale down. Now we'll do some sweeping breaths as you inhale. Arms sweep up and out, lift up nice and tall, as you exhale relax the arms down. Again inhale, and exhale down. Let's do one more. Open up. Inhale, and exhale.

Let's bring your hands together behind your back, fingers interlaced, lift up your chest and chin and open up the front of your body, lift yourself up. Create a stretch through the chest, through the throat. Shoulder blades pulled together, strengthening the middle of the back. Just breathe here, opening up the front of your body, creating expansiveness. And then exhale, relax your arms, shake them out.

Let's do a couple of exercises to focus on strength and balance. We'll do some squats, lifting the arms out to the sides. If you're seated you'll focus on the arm exercise. If you're standing, your feet are hip-width apart. We're going to inhale and center our body, exhale feeling nice and grounded. Now we'll just breathe naturally as we do our squats. Bend at the knees, belly button back to the spine, tailbone's tucked under. Knees about at the toes; you don't want to go past the toes, that puts the knees at risk. Keep the knees at the toes. Chest stays lifted. You're not scrunching; you're staying nice and tall here. You're going to lift your arms out to the side, and we're going to hold a count of five here, breathing in and out. Feeling strong through the legs, stretching out through the arms, and then inhale come up. Exhale bending down, arms come up. Again if you're working from a seated position, you're working the arms, and focusing on strong posture, engaging the core of your body. Exhale come back up. If it starts to get easy, you can even add some light hand weights. Bending down into your squat, hold here for a count of 5, 4, 3, 2, 1. And relax. We're going to take two more, coming into your squat, feel the strength of your glutes, your thighs. Breathe into it. And relax. One more. Come into your squat, hold it here. You want a slightly different challenge, try lifting your toes off the ground, feeling how that changes your weight and your balance and engages your quadriceps a little bit more. Then relax; shake your legs out.

Let's take a few balance exercises now to engage your core-body muscles. Let's stand beside the chair, right foot beside the chair, right hand on the back of the chair for support. You'll start with your weight on your right foot. The chair is here to support you as needed. You'll bend the left knee, and just bring the left hand to the left ankle. This is called stork pose. If you're feeling nice and solid here, you can bring the hand to the hip. If you're seated, you'll be a little bit forward on the chair, and bring the leg up behind you as well, so you're stretching the front of the leg, opening it up. If you're standing and you're solid with your balance, hands on the hip. If you're feeling comfortable you can bring the arm up beside you. If you need to go back to the chair that's OK. It's more challenging to balance when you're in shoes. That's why yoga classes are usually done barefoot. Your foot can engage with the floor. Again, balancing, solid, arm is up, if you'd like to challenge yourself further you can take it to dancer pose. Arm out in front of you, foot coming behind you. Focus your gaze at one point to find your stability. Then when you're done you bring the foot down and the hand down. Again, weight solid on the right foot, start with the chair for balance, bring the left knee up in front of you. Hand comes to the waist, and if you're feeling solid, both hands at the waist. If you're seated, again forward on the chair, lift the left foot up, engaging the muscles of the leg to strengthen them. Balance here whether you're standing or seated. And then relax the leg down.

We'll take the other side, so if you're seated, slightly forward and to the side on the chair. We'll start with stork pose, bend the right knee behind you, you can hold the ankle if that feels comfortable. Stretching the front of the leg. If you're standing, now your left side is beside the chair, left hand on the chair, weight on the left foot. Bend the right knee back. If you're feeling comfortable, take the ankle in your hand. You're feeling solid, hand comes to the waist. Or up beside you. If you want to challenge it further you move to dancer. Forward through the arm, back through the leg, focus your gaze at one point that helps you find your stability and your balance, and then when you're ready come back to center, release the hand and the foot. We'll try it forward now, hand starts at the chair, lift the right knee in front of you. Hand comes to the waist if you're feeling comfortable, and if you're seated, you've got the right leg lifted up, engaging the muscles of the thigh. Nice, tall posture whether you're seated or standing, working on your core-body strength. And then release the leg.

We're going to do a couple of pelvic floor exercises here. Nice, wide legs. Toes are turned out. Sit up tall, lift your chest, center your posture. We're going to do a couple of pelvic floor exercises here to strengthen the pelvic floor, make sure that we're working on that part of our body as well. Focus your awareness at your pelvic floor, and then lift up and hold there for 5, 4, 3, 2, 1 and relax. Remember to keep your thighs, stomach, and bottom soft; we're isolating the muscles of the pelvic floor. Contract up and hold for 5, 4, 3, 2, 1, release. Again lift it up and hold for 5, 4, 3, 2, 1, release. Again contract and hold for 5, 4, 3, 2, 1, release. One more, contract and hold for 5, 4, 3, 2, 1, release. Relax your hands; fold your body forward between your legs, relaxing down into a forward bend. Let your hands soften between your legs. Let your head sink down. Take a couple of deep breaths here. Just let your body relax into the forward bend. Then bring your hands to your knees.

Use your hands to push yourself back up to sitting, back up to center. Bring your legs back together, hands onto your stomach.

We'll start with some deep breathing. As you inhale, breathe in a nice deep breath. Let the lower lobes of your stomach expand but your stomach relax out into your hands. As you exhale, belly button back to the spine, pushing the air out of your body. Inhale, stomach expands, breath fills your body. Exhale, belly button back to the spine. This time once you've pushed all the air out of your body we're going to take stomach pump; contract your stomach back and forth, engaging the muscles of your abdomen. Inhale, exhale all the way out, and stomach pump, contract, engage your abdominal muscles, use your core. Inhale, exhale, and pump your stomach. While you're pumping, you're not breathing, you're focusing on your core-body muscles. Inhale, exhale all the way out, belly button back to the spine. One more time, contract back and forth, pump your stomach muscles. And then relax. Come back to a centered awareness with your palms open on your lap. Take a few deep breaths here, exhaling away any stress or tension, inhaling in energy and renewal for your day. Feel a sense of accomplishment for making your health a priority in your busy schedule. A little bit counts, and you just made every minute count in your health. Great work.

Manage Stress (10 minutes)

It's been one of those days. Nothing's going right. You just want to go back to bed and hide under the covers. Or maybe you feel like biting a few people's heads off. Let's put that negative energy to good use and channel it into your health and well-being. The first thing we're going to do is shake off the stress, using some yoga and Qigong energy exercises. If you prefer to stay seated, you can still do the workout.

We'll start with yoga jelly pose. Whether you're seated or standing, you're going to bring your arms up and you're going to shake your whole body. You're going to shake side to side, and you're going to shake forward and backward. Feel silly, laugh if you want, but just move. Shake. Move your whole body and shake, shake, shake to get that energy out. What we're trying to do is process the adrenaline and stress hormones that flood your body when you're stressed, angry, or frustrated. The best way to use them is to move. Shake a little bit more. And then relax, and we're going to do a Qigong exercise called making rain.

You can be standing, or you can be seated in a nice comfortable posture. Either way you're going to float your arms up to shoulder height, straight out in front of you. Fingers are soft, dangling down. Gently allow your whole body to become soft. You'll slowly just shake down as if you're letting rain come out of your fingertips. Allow your breath to be soft and natural and imagine that all the stress in your body is raining out of your fingertips, leaving your body softer, more relaxed. Continue to gently, softly shake the stress out of your body, letting it drip out of your fingertips. Then relax, and straighten your legs out if you're standing, come back to a comfortable seated position if you're seated. We'll work the tension out. Usually we hold most of the tension in our shoulders and our neck.

We'll do some neck stretches here. Right ear to your right shoulder, nice long stretch, press it down through the heel of your left hand to open up the side of the neck. Close your eyes and we'll take a couple of breaths here just relaxing into that, feeling yourself open up that shoulder. Then take the left ear to the left shoulder; press down through the hell of your right hand. Close your eyes; sink into that stretch, opening up the neck. Breathing in and out through the nose. And back to center. We're going to look to the right; keep the left shoulder back so you're opening up the side of the neck. Nice, long stretch. Again, close your eyes, take your awareness within. Back to center; look to the left side. And back to center. Look up, nice long stretch, opening up the front of the throat. And then tuck the chin in, opening up the back of the neck, creating space between the shoulder blades. Back up to center.

We're going to take some shoulder shrugs. Give yourself a little massage. Squeeze your shoulders all the way up. Exhale, take them down. Inhale, squeeze them up. Exhale, take them down. Inhale, squeeze. Exhale, take them down. Now let's roll the shoulders backward. You might hear some clicking; that's OK, that's normal. Just roll gentle range of motion through the shoulders, rolling backwards. Open up the chest. And then relax. Now let's take your right arm across, bring your left hand to the upper arm and help stretch that arm across the front of your body. Opening up the shoulder. Couple of deep breaths here, really feel your shoulder open up. And then relax that. Take the other side. Left arm across, right hand to the upper arm, nice long stretch. And then release that down.

Interlace your fingers, bring your hands behind your head, pull your elbows out, opening your chest up. We'll stay here for a couple of deep breaths; close your eyes, feel yourself pulling your shoulder blades together to strengthen the middle of the back. Open up the chest, breathe here. Now let's stretch to the left, pulling the left elbow down. Right elbow up. Keep pulling back through the elbows, though, to keep the chest open. And then up to center, exhale the other side, right elbow down, left elbow up, pull back through the elbows to keep the chest open. And back up to center, release the arms shake them out.

Now that we've shaken out the stress and worked out some of that tension. Let's build some strong positive energy. We're going to take warrior 1. This is a pose that's great for helping you to feel centered and ground. If you're standing, step your right foot back a little bit. Turn the toes out gently just to about 2 o'clock if you were standing on a clock face. Step the left foot forward into a lunge, bending that knee. The knee should be aligned with the heel of the foot, so that the knee is protected. Square your hips forward to the front leg. If you need to, you can hold onto the chair for support, and you're going to stretch your arms up, looking up between your fingertips. If you're seated, you're gonna come to the front of your chair and just ground that front leg, tuck the right leg behind you a little bit to open up the front of that thigh, and the arms are up, you're looking up between your hands. You can be seated or standing; either way, your gaze is looking upward, your posture is tall, you're opening the front of your body to create strength, to create expansiveness, to feel strong and centered and positive. Couple more breaths here. And then exhale the arms down, step your feet together. We'll take the other side. Again, you can use the chair for support with one hand. You can do it seated or standing, whatever feels comfortable to you. Right foot's forward, left foot's back, turned in a little bit. If you were on a clock face this time it's 10 o'clock with the back toes.

The front knee's bent, knee over the ankle, arms sweep up, nice and tall, gaze is up, you're lifting the front of your body, creating openness and stretch. If you're seated, again the back leg is tucked in, open that front leg, front knee is forward, arms are up and you're lifting upward, creating strength and openness in your body. Breathe into your warrior pose a couple of breaths here. Then relax your arms, bring your feet back to center. You're standing, step your feet back together.

We're going to come to sitting on the chair now. We're going to take what's called lion pose. Lion pose is about feeling strong and fierce. It's got some sound to it because you're working to open up your chest and throat, so if you're in your office or your cubicle and it's a quiet space, skip the sound effects, just do the pose. If you've got the space, actually make the vocalization to feel strength building in your voice and your body and your energy. You're going to place your feet nice and solid, knees are about hip-width apart. Heels of the hands come onto the knees. You're going to push your chest forward between your arms, opening up the front of the body. Lift your chin to open your throat, so nice, long open line from the belly button up to the chin. Open your mouth nice and wide. You're going to stick your tongue out and you're going to stretch your whole body as you growl through it. [Growl.] So a nice growl as you're stretching and opening. Let's take one more, really open up. [Growl.] Feel your voice creating strength in your body. Try one more, you take the sound this time. And then relax that, come back to a comfortable seated position on your chair.

We're going to take the positive energy within now. We're going to spread the legs nice and wide, hands on knees, and we're going to take a forward bend, bringing this energy within us. Fold forward between your legs, relax your head down. Let yourself sink into your forward bend. Then bring your hands to your knees, push yourself back up to sitting. Bring your legs back together, your palms are open on your lap, close your eyes, and let's just take a couple of deep breaths here, breathing in a sense of strength and energy, feeling strong and brave and relaxed. Exhale away any stress or tension. Inhale in. Exhale out. One more breath, inhale. And exhale. Feel ready to take on any challenge in front of you, and face the day with a renewed sense of who you are and all that you can accomplish.

Get Energized (10 minutes)

You didn't sleep well last night, or life got busy and you didn't get much sleep. So you're feeling tired, a little sluggish. Let's help you breathe deeper and find some energy from within to help you get through the day. We'll start in a comfortable seated position on a chair.

Your posture is open yet relaxed, shoulders rolled down and back, palms open in your lap. We'll take a few gentle breaths to bring your energy and attention within. Close your eyes, breathing in and out through the nose, take a nice deep inhalation, breathing into the lower lobes of the lungs, letting the stomach soften and relax. As you exhale, push the belly button back towards the spine and exhale all the way out, contracting the abdomen to push the air out of your body. Again inhale, and exhale. Belly button back to the spine, air pushes out of your body. Inhale deeply, exhale all the way out. Taking nice, deep, gentle breaths, as you inhale breathing in a sense of being centered, peaceful, calm. As you exhale, breathing out the fatigue, breathing out the stress, breathing out the sense of being tired. Inhaling in energy one more time, and exhale all the way out.

Now we'll take a kundalini twist, which is a great exercise to energize your internal organs, your body moving, your blood flowing. Bring your arms up, elbows are bent fingers spread wide, and we'll twist from the waist back and forth. If you're comfortable close your eyes, take your focus within and just feel yourself moving, creating energy in your body with movement. Breathing naturally and gently through the nose. Couple more twists here. And then come on back to center, relax your hands down.

We're going to take a breathing exercise now called breath of fire. This is a great exercise for energizing your body and your mind. If you have a history of high blood pressure or panic attacks, though, skip this one and just continue breathing gently and normally. You're gonna curl your fingers into your palms with your thumbs extended and then sweep your arms up and out from your shoulders to form a Y. Take a nice deep breath, and then we're going to take fast, panting breaths through the nose. You're breathing like a dog in the summer heat, contracting your stomach muscles as you breathe. Inhale, and then pant. Now stretch up a little bit more through the arms, lengthen out through the thumbs, one more time. Inhale, and pant. Relax your hands down.

Now we're going to try a downward facing dog pose standing beside the chair. I'll also show you a seated modification if you prefer to stay seated. If you're comfortable stand on up, come beside your chair, facing the side of your chair. Step back a little bit, place your hands in the center of your chair. Then you're going to step your feet back, walk your fingers forward, push back through your hips and relax your head down between your arms. You're creating a nice long stretch from the top of your head to the base of your spine, creating length in the stretch. If you're seated, come to the edge of the chair. Feet are nice and wide. Fold your body forward so that your chest is on your thighs. Stretch out through your fingertips. Again, head between your arms, stretching long between your fingertips, so that you create space from the top of your head to the base of the spine. What we're doing is opening up the spine, creating some length, whether you're stretching seated, or standing, we're creating a nice, long open stretch in the body, improving blood flow and energy flow in your spine. Take a couple more deep breaths here. Just relax into it. Really stretch back, stretch forward through the fingertips, create length, nice breaths here, in and out through the nose. Remember to breathe. If you're standing, you're going to just walk forward to the chair, gently push yourself up. If you're seated, put your hands on your knees and push your body back up. If you're standing we're going to stay standing; if you're seated, that's fine. Either way, nice good posture. If you're standing, feet are wide, chest open, hands relaxed beside you. If you're seated, again shoulders rolled down and back, nice open posture.

We're going to take some arm-sweeping breaths, 10 breaths. Inhale up, touch your hands up at the top. Exhale down. Inhale, breathe, exhale down. Inhale up, exhale. Inhale up, exhale. Inhale, exhale. Inhale, exhale. Inhale, exhale. Inhale, exhale. Two more. Inhale, exhale. And inhale, reach up tall, open up your body, and exhale down. Now inhale your arms up again, interlace your fingers, stretch your index finger and your thumb up, and we're going to stretch to the left side, lengthening up through the right side of the body. Nice, long stretch whether you're standing or seated, you're doing the same stretch here to lengthen, breathe into it, feel yourself opening up your torso.

Then back to center, take a nice inhale. And exhale other side, nice long stretch. Let's do one more. Come back up to center, inhale. Exhale left, nice long stretch. Inhale up to center. Exhale to the other side, nice long stretch. Inhale center, exhale, relax your arms. Shake your arms out if you need to.

We're going to take an eagle pose. This is a balancing pose that works the whole body. I'll show it standing first and then I'll show the chair modification if you're remaining seated. You're beside the chair; chair's here for balance if you need it. Put your weight on your left foot, cross your right leg over the left. Then you're going to tuck that right foot behind your left ankle. If you're feeling comfortable there, and you can, you're going to let go of the chair, cross your arms, and then bring the forward arm around to bring your palms together. If you're seated, very similar. You're going to cross one leg over, try to tuck the toe behind the calf, cross one arm over and then bring that hand around so that you bring your palms together. You'll feel a great stretch through the upper arms, through the back, also through the hips and legs. Eagle pose is great for circulation in the legs. Yoga theory holds that it actually helps prevent or improve the condition of varicose veins. If you're feeling comfortable with your balance, and you're standing, you can try to sink into it. Bring your elbow down onto your knee, just pause here. Focus your gaze at one point, that helps with your balance. If you lose your balance, no big deal, just pick it up and try again. Then when you're ready to come up, gently come up, unwind, unwrap.

Let's take the other side. This time weight's on the right foot, crossing the left foot over. Same thing if you're seated, crossing the left leg over. Then you're going to tuck the left toe behind. Opposite arm so this time right arm on bottom, left arm on top, bring the left hand around the front. Then if your balance is good, you're feeling comfortable, bring your elbows down to your knees. Focus your gaze at one point. Breathe into it. And then when you're ready, come on up, unwrap, unwind.

We're going to take a mountain pose to center our awareness. If you're standing, feet are hip-width apart, toes gently turned in, heels gently open, grounding into the floor. If you're seated, nice good posture, feet planted, chest open, arms beside you. Solid posture, plant your feet into the earth, roll your shoulders down and back. Palms are open beside you. Focus your awareness on being strong, on connecting through the soles of your feet. Close your eyes and take a few more deep breaths. Really breathe into your lungs. Bring oxygen into your body. Charge yourself with energy, vitality, refreshment. Nice, deep, strong breath here. Remember, whenever you feel tired, stop and take five deep breaths to recharge and renew. Have an energetic day!

Chair Yoga
Lecture 17

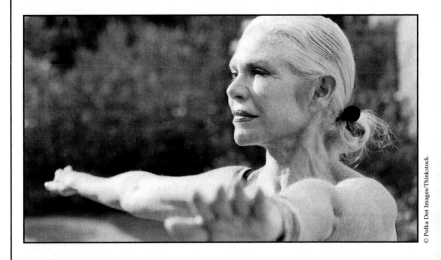

© Polka Dot Images/Thinkstock.

Yoga is a mindful fitness practice that combines physical exercises with breathing exercises and deliberate mental focus. Chair yoga provides an adapted yoga workout to ensure that the benefits of yoga are accessible to everyone. You've likely seen images of yoga in the mass media that make it look complicated, unusual, and even stressful. But as you'll see in this session, yoga can be a simple practice and a comfortable form of physical exercise. At the end of the session, you should set an intention to maintain the sense of control and peace gained through yoga practice.

Suggested Reading

International Association of Yoga Therapists, http://www.iayt.org/.

Yee, *Yoga*.

Yoga Alliance, https://www.yogaalliance.org/.

Yoga Journal, http://www.yogajournal.com/.

Chair Yoga
Lecture 17—Transcript

Chair Yoga (35 minutes)

Yoga is a mindful fitness practice that combines physical exercise with focused breathing and deliberate mental focus. Chair yoga provides an adapted yoga workout to offer the benefits of yoga, which is accessible for everyone, and which you can do anywhere. The chair is for balance and support, both for those who stand to do these exercises and for those who prefer, for whatever reason, to remain seated. You will benefit from these exercises whether you choose to stay seated or stand.

To begin, come into a comfortable seated position on a chair. Feet are slightly apart, and gently pressing into the floor. Palms are open on your lap, shoulders rolled down and back to open up your chest, chin tucks in lightly to create space at the back of the neck. Close your eyes, and take your attention within.

We'll start with a few minutes of breathing exercises. Bring your awareness to your nose, and take an inhalation through the nose, and bringing the breath into your body, into the lower lobes of your lungs, letting your stomach soften and relax as you inhale. As you exhale, belly button back to the spine, releasing the air out of your body, feeling stress dissolve out as you exhale. Inhale, and exhale. Inhale, exhale. Soft, deliberate, focused breathing. Inhale, exhale. Inhale, exhale. Continue breathing throughout this practice, being deliberate and focused with your breaths, breathing in and out through your nose. Remembering to breathe through your nose helps you to control your breath, helps you to keep a sense of centeredness, focused awareness in your breath, remembering not to take the breath for granted.

Let's work on opening up the neck now. We'll start with a nice relaxed neck, nice relaxed shoulders. We're going to take the right ear towards the right shoulder. Press down through the heel of your left hand. Close your eyes if you can. Take your attention within. Stretch through the side of the neck, feel it opening up. Couple deep breaths here; each breath feeling your muscles soften and relax. Now back to center, let's take the other side. Press down through the heel of the right hand, left ear towards the shoulder. And come on back to center. Now let's look over the right shoulder. Try to keep your left shoulder where it is so that you're really opening up the side of the neck. We can hold a lot of tension in our throats; we can get very jammed up when we're stressed, so it's good to open up the neck, open up the throat. Let yourself relax and release that stress. Deep breaths here. And come back to center. Let's take it the other direction. Nice, long stretch, breathing into it. And back to center. Let's tuck the chin all the way in, lengthening the back of the neck, creating space at the base of the head, breathe here. It's very easy to forget to breathe; really use that as a way to focus your attention, focus your awareness.

Back to center and then keep your shoulders down, lift your chin as much as you can to open up the front of the throat, create space in the front of your body. We spend so much time hunched over keyboards and steering wheels, it's good to open up the front to create space and expansion. Come on back to center. We're going to bring your hands onto your knees and we're going to take some spinal rolls. As you inhale, press your hands into your knees and lift your chest, lift your chin, look up, lengthen the front of your body. As you exhale, tuck your chin in, roll your spine. As you inhale, lift, open. As you exhale, roll and tuck in. Inhale lift. Exhale roll. Inhale lift. Exhale roll. Again close your eyes; take your focus inward. Inhale lift; exhale roll. Inhale lift; exhale roll. One more inhale. And exhale. Back up to center.

Keep your hands on your knees. We're going to take some rolling movement from the waist to open up your torso. As you exhale, we're going to fold forward; as you begin to inhale we're going to roll over towards the right, come up, and exhale down around the other side. Inhaling as you come up, exhaling as you fold forward. Close your eyes as soon as you feel comfortable and just take soft, gentle movement through the waist, breathing through the nose. Inhaling up, exhaling down. Elbows are gently out to the side; let your body feel comfortable as you move. Inhaling up, exhaling down. The next time we get up to the top we're going to switch directions. Exhale forward, inhale up. Close your eyes again when you feel comfortable. Moving gently. Exhale forward. Inhale up. And come on back up to center.

Bring your left hand to the outside of your right knee, right hand behind you to the chair. Gently twist to look over the shoulder. Your hand on the chair is wherever you feel comfortable; it might be up high, it might be down low. Listen to what feels good for your shoulder. You'll start gently with the twist through your upper body, through your chest. You might just be looking a little bit over your chest. If you're feeling very comfortable, you can rotate back over the shoulder. The twist should originate through your torso and your upper body. The head and neck turn because of the movement of your upper body. Keep the head and the neck natural, relaxed, soft. Breathe into it. Twists are very good for your waist; they're good for moving circulation through your torso. Breathe here for a couple of breaths, feel that you can sink into the twist a little bit deeper as you breathe into it. And exhale come on back to center.

Let's take the other side. Right hand to the outside of the left knee; left hand to the chair behind you, using the hand against the knee to help you rotate. Lifting through the chest, keep your body open and lifted as you twist. You'll feel it through your low back, the middle of your back, your hips. Breathe into it. Again, when you feel comfortable, close your eyes, take your focus within. Couple more breaths here. And exhale, come on back to center.

We're going to do an arm exercise now, so you're going to take your arms straight out from your shoulders. This seems very simple but we're going to do it for a little bit. You're just gently going to start moving your arms up and down, breathing while you're here. In the beginning it seems like not much exercise at all, but this is really an exercise in patience, and in focus, and in being very deliberate because as you begin to move you'll start to become more aware of your arms. They'll start to feel heavier. But if they start to hurt, distract yourself by using this time to think of something you've accomplished and how you were successful in that. Or, think about something you are worried about and set an intention that you know you will be successful at that. Part of yoga is learning that you can do what you set out to do. It's about learning that you're strong, that you're powerful, that you're capable. That by being centered within yourself you have the capacity to do warrior poses, which we'll do later today, to continue moving your arms even when they hurt and you feel like you just want to stop, to focus your awareness and breathe even when you feel stressed and feel your mind racing in a million different directions. That's a big part of what yoga is, is learning that you have the capacity to control your mind, to control your breathing, to control your body, to control what you're doing and how you feel. You learn that sense of centered capability. Couple more breaths here, breathing through the discomfort in your arms, feeling that strong sense of accomplishment for pushing through, and then exhale, relax your arms down, shake them out.

We'll come now to standing to take mountain pose. In standing we'll start in mountain pose, a foundational yoga posture, to help you work on balance and stability. Feet are about hip-width apart; toes are turned in just slightly. Bring one hand to your ribcage, one hand to your tailbone, tuck your ribs in and your tailbone under to align your spine. Release your hands beside you; roll your shoulders down and back, tuck your chin in. Back of the neck is long. If you're seated, you can continue with your posture while seated to work on upper body. Eyes are closed if you feel comfortable, but notice that your balance is more challenged when your eyes are closed. Feel a sense of being solid and grounded, feeling your weight pressed down through your feet, anchoring you into the ground beneath you. Feel a sense of being stable. Strong. Sturdy. Again, if you're seated focus on pressing your feet into the ground beneath you, keeping your chest open, your spine long. Working on posture whether you're standing or sitting right now, feeling strong, stable, solid. One more nice deep breath here, in and out through the nose. And then open up your eyes, relax your legs a little bit.

In our lecture on fitness fundamentals, we talked about the importance of building balance and muscular flexibility and strength. These are all central components of what we do in yoga. The first thing we'll do are some side stretches. Feet are nice and wide. Inhale, lift your right arm up, long over your left side. Look up towards your middle fingertip if you feel comfortable. Again, breathing in and out through the nose, slow and deliberate in your breath. Now exhale it down. Inhale up the left arm, looking up at the middle fingertip, nice long stretch. And exhale down. We'll take it a little bit more fluidly. Inhale lift, exhale down. Other side, inhale lift, exhale down. Inhale lift and stretch, lengthen, exhale down. Inhale lift and stretch, exhale down. One more set, inhale. Exhale. Inhale. Exhale.

We're going to take a warrior pose now, coming beside the chair. Turn your toes in towards your chair; your left foot steps back. Arch of the foot aligned with the heel of the right foot, toes turned in slightly. Bend in toward the right knee. Bring your left hand to your left hip, your right hand to your bottom, pulling your hip back and your bottom slightly forward to open up your pelvis. Right knee towards the little-toe side of the foot to strengthen the inner thigh. If you're comfortable, arms are straight out through your shoulders, gaze focused at your middle fingertip. If you need support you can hold on to the side of your chair; if you're seated you can follow along with your upper body, working on strength, posture, and balance. Focus your gaze at your middle fingertip. Feel a sense of being very strong. We'll take several deep breaths here as we do our warrior pose. There's a whole series of warrior poses in yoga, all of them focused on strength of the internal body. It's very interesting because in the U.S. we have this notion that yoga is a woman's practice, but originally, in India, men were the ones who practiced yoga, and women were not allowed to. In fact, the warrior component stems from some ancient writings in the Bhagavad Gita.

Let's go ahead and move to the other side. Relax your arms; straighten your legs, shake them out. Walk around to the other side and again, left toes towards the chair, right toes turned in slightly. Back of the heel aligned with the arch of the foot, bend into the front knee, open up the pelvis. As you get more comfortable and strong, you can walk that back leg back further to work more on strength of the lower body. Arms are out at the shoulders or holding on to the back of the chair if you feel more comfortable. Focus your gaze on that middle fingertip, and feel strong here in your warrior pose. In the Bhagavad Gita, some of the early writings about yoga actually take place in the context of a battlefield conversation. In a fluid sense of continuity, there are doctors and researchers in the VA medical system who have found that yoga is very helpful for soldiers dealing with combat-related conditions such as post-traumatic stress disorder. Feel one more deep stretch. And release your arms. If you need to use the chair that's perfectly fine. Step your feet together, shake your legs out.

We're going to take a triangle pose now, so you'll come centered with the chair, left toes under. Right foot is back. Again, heal aligned with the arch of the foot. If you're seated, working with the arms and upper body. Arms are straight out of the shoulders. Start by bringing the right hand to your right hip, and as if you were a teapot, bend yourself over at the waist. Bring your hand onto the chair, and then lift that right arm up straight out of the shoulder. If it's comfortable for your neck you can look up at the middle fingertip. If that hurts your neck you can look down at the middle fingertip of the bottom hand. If you're comfortable here with your stretch and you want to take it further, you can bring your hand down onto your shin, but you don't want to sink into the shin. You want to stay lifted. Just using the hand gently there as a place of support. Try to rotate the top hip back, feel a sense of stretching, elongation through the upper body. Breathe into it. Inhale up. Relax your arms down. Let's take it on the other side.

Right toes under, left foot stepped back nice and wide, torso centered, arms out. Again, I'm a little teapot, tip yourself over. Stretch the arm up. If you're feeling comfortable you can take that lower hand down. Nice, long stretch. You'll feel a stretch through the inner thighs, through the back hip. Lifting up through the ribcage. Remember to breathe. It's very easy to accidentally hold your breath. Inhale up; step your feet together; shake your arms and legs out.

We're going to take tree pose now, which is a balanced pose to work on stability of the core body, strength of the legs. We'll build from the ground up, helping you to find the sense of balance that's comfortable for you. If you're seated, follow along with the upper body, and you can still work your feet at the floor. Start with your right hand on the chair for support. Weight on the right foot. Bring your left foot to the ankle with your toes on the floor. If that feels comfortable and you want to take it a little bit farther, you can bring the foot up to the inside of the shin, knee stretching out to the side. If that's still feeling comfortable, you can bring the foot up inside the thigh, but not at the knee, never at the knee—the knee is very fragile. So we either go above or below the knee. If you're feeling solid here, bring one hand and then the other together in front of your chest. You'll wobble a little bit; that's normal, it's OK. Focus your awareness; you've focused your gaze on one point. That fixed gaze will help you be much more stable and steady. If you're feeling comfortable, arms up over your head. Breathe here. If you lose your balance, that's OK, you pick it up and you try again. On your next breath exhale your arms out, relax the foot, shake it out.

We'll come to the other side to take tree on the other side. Weight starts on the left foot, toes start on the ground, knee turned out. This is a great stretch, a great balancing pose, even if you stay here so work with what feels comfortable for your body. Go at the pace that feels good for you. It's all about the internal practice so focus on that sense of staying internal, staying comfortable, challenging yourself in a safe way. If you're feeling comfortable and ready, you can bring the foot up to the inside of the shin. If that still feels comfortable you can bring up inside the thigh, but again, never the knee. You can bring one hand up if that's solid. If you're still feeling stable, the other hand comes up. You may wobble; it's OK, grab the chair. Find your sense of balance. Reestablish your stability. Bring your arms up if you're feeling comfortable. If you're seated, bring your arms up, focus on lifting up through the upper body. Couple more breaths here. Again, if you lose your balance just pick it up and start over again. And exhale, release the arms, release the foot, shake the legs out.

We're going to take big toe series now, which is a strengthening series for the lower body, the legs in particular. You might start with a hand on the chair if that feels comfortable; hand is on the hip. We'll start with the weight on the left leg. If you're seated, you'll be working the legs from a seated position. Lifting the right foot out in front of you to work on strengthening the quadriceps, your glutes, your core body. If you're feeling comfortable with your balance, bring your other hand to your hip. If you waver go back to the chair, that's OK. Be patient with your body. Feel a sense of stability here, ground through the feet.

Relax that foot, let's take the other side, weight solid on the right toe. Lift the left leg. If you're feeling comfortable, lift the leg up a little higher, challenging the quadriceps a little bit more. Release it down, shake your legs out. Again, starting with the hand at the back of the chair, bend the right knee. Bring your right hand to your right knee. If you're solid, bring your left hand to your hip. Focus on strengthening through the leg, pressing the left foot into the ground beneath you to feel solid and stable. If you're comfortable, open the right knee out to the side. If you're really feeling good about your balance try looking over your left shoulder. If you need to, you can hold onto the chair for support, listen to what's comfortable for your body. Then bring the knee and your gaze back to center, release the foot, shake it out. Bring your left hand to the chair again and let's lift the right leg out to the side, lifting through the glutes, through the side of the leg. If you're solid both hands to the hips. Breathe. And then release that leg, and shake the legs out.

Let's take the other side. Again, right hand starts on the back of the chair, left hand on the hip. Bring the left knee up. If you're comfortable, left hand to the knee. If you're still feeling solid, right hand comes to the hip. If it feels hard to do, or seems like you're not doing well, don't worry about it. Just focus on improvement, focus on how you feel inside. It doesn't matter how it looks; yoga's not a spectator sport. It's all about how you feel inside. If you're feeling solid, that left knee goes out to the side. If you're ready to challenge your balance a little bit more, take your gaze over the right shoulder. Gaze and the knee back to the center, relax the hand and foot. Shake your legs out. Again, hand to the back of the chair, let's lift the left leg out to the side, torso's nice and tall. If you're comfortable, both hands to the hips. Keep your mind focused, your breath controlled. And then release that leg. Shake it out. Shake out the arms.

Come back to the front of your chair again for space, and we're going to take star pose. Feet are nice and wide, arms stretch out through the shoulders through the fingertips, lift the top of your head. Open your body in five directions like a star, and really stretch and expand. Close your eyes if you feel comfortable. Take a nice deep inhalation. As you exhale, breathe out completely, stretching out through the fingertips, up through the top of the head. Couple more deep breaths, really open. Star pose is a great pose when you're in the middle of the day and you're in that midafternoon slump and you're feeling tired to just stand up and open your body in five directions and create expansion and openness. Couple more deep breaths. Then exhale, release your arms, step your feet together, shake your legs out and we're going to come back to sitting on the chair.

We'll take a seated forward bend now so come to the front of your chair, spread your legs nice and wide, toes are turned out. Nice alignment from the hip to the knee to the ankles. Hands start gently on your knees, and we're going to take a nice inhalation. As you exhale, fold your body forward between your legs, let your hands relax down to your feet, let your head relax down between your legs. Just sink into your forward bend; relax here.

Forward bends are great for taking your energy within. If you're feeling stressed, if the world's feeling a little overwhelming, if everything's too busy or rushed, just take a forward bend. Focus yourself within. Breathe into it. In and out through the nose, a couple more gentle breaths. Let your neck release down, gentle traction for your neck to relax it. Release any stress or tension out of the back of your neck, the back of your head. Then when you're ready to come up, bring your hands to your knees and use your hands to press yourself up, bringing yourself up gently.

Bring your feet back together, and we'll take a camel pose. You're going to start with your hips to knees to ankles in a nice straight line, feet about hip-width apart. Sitting nice and tall, bring your hands behind you, low on your chair, and lift your chest and chin. Open up the front of your body. Strengthening the muscles of the back, expanding the muscles of the chest. Breathe here. If you're feeling comfortable and you want to take it a little bit farther, bring your hands into fists. Place them at your lower back, right about hip height. Pull your elbows back, lift your chest and chin, push your back forward with your fists. Camel pose is a great one for opening up the front of the body. Breathe here; remember to take nice, slow, deliberate breaths in and out through the nose. And then come back up to center.

We're going to stretch the fingers, the hands and the feet, working on opening up the joints. We're going to take the hands straight out in front of us. Sit back on the chair so you can lift your legs up too. We're going to stretch the toes, stretch the fingers nice and wide, open them up, and then curl them in. As you inhale, open them up; as you exhale, curl them all in. As you inhale open them up; as you exhale curl them all in. This is great if you've got arthritis in your joints to keep movement in your hands and feet. Inhale, open, stretch as wide as you can. Exhale, curl them in, squeeze them in tight. If you feel comfortable being silly, you want to try one more extension, you can work with your face while you're going your hands and feet. You can open up wide, and then scrunch everything in tight. Great for working through the stressors in your face. Open wide. Curl in tight. It's good to laugh at yourself, good to be OK with being silly. Open up wide, curl everything in tight. And then relax. Release it down. Come back into comfortable seated position. Place your palms open on your lap. Come back into nice posture, shoulders rolled down and back, chin is tucked in, back of the neck is long.

Always come back to those fundamental components of your posture: open chest, belly button towards the spine, tailbone tucked under, nice solid posture. Close your eyes and take a nice inhalation and exhale all the way out. Breathing again in and out through the nose, focusing your awareness, focusing your mind, inhale in, exhale out. Inhale, exhale. Breathe in a sense of being center, calm, stable. Exhale away any residual stress or tension. Inhale in a sense of being strong and healthy and well. Exhale away any pain or discomfort. Feel how strong and healthy you are. Inhale. Exhale. Couple more deep breaths. Then gently open your eyes. Just stay seated here for a moment and become aware of how you are feeling. Is your mind a little calmer? Are your shoulders a little looser? Is your breathing a little quieter?

You've likely seen images of yoga in the mass media which make it look complicated, unusual, and even stressful. But as you experienced in this session, yoga can be a simple practice and a comfortable form of physical exercise which incorporates focused attention and deliberate breathing to bring about relaxation. I'd like you to take a moment now to set an intention. Setting an intention helps you transition the gains you've made during the yoga session to the rest of your day. It helps you form the connection between your yoga and your life, allowing you to integrate yoga as more than just physical exercise.

Let's do that now. Take another deep breath, inhaling deeply. Now exhale completely. Breathing gently, set an intention to maintain the sense of calm and quiet that you feel right now. Set an intention to become more aware and more deliberate about how you react to stressors. Set an intention to remember that you can purposefully modify your response to stress, to life through calm, quiet breathing and gentle exercise. Set an intention to maintain a sense of control and peace throughout the rest of your day.

The Sanskrit word *Namaste* is the traditional ending for a yoga practice. It means that the good in me recognizes the good in you. Thank you for sharing your goodness with me today in the practice of yoga. *Namaste*.

Qigong—Practicing Fluid Movement
Lecture 18

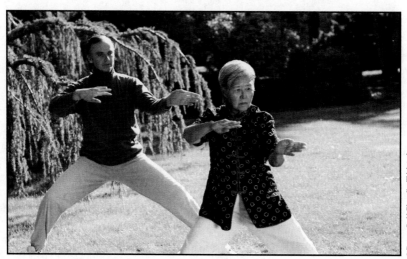

© Duncan Smith/Photodisc/Thinkstock.

Tai Chi and Qigong are mindful fitness practices that focus on slow, deliberate movement integrated with breathing exercises. These practices are uniquely suited to improve balance and stability, improve posture, and increase lung capacity. They are built on two philosophical premises: encouraging the healthy flow of energy (*qi*) through the body and encouraging the balance of opposing forces (yin and yang) within the body.

Suggested Reading

American Tai Chi and Qigong Association, http://www.americantaichi.org/about.asp.

Cohen, *The Way of Qigong*.

National Qigong Association, http://www.nqa.org.

Wayne, *The Harvard Medical School Guide to Tai Chi*.

Qigong—Practicing Fluid Movement
Lecture 18—Transcript

Qigong: Practicing Fluid Movement (30 minutes)

Tai Chi and Qigong are mindful fitness practices that focus on slow, deliberate movement integrated with breathing exercises. Tai Chi and Qigong are uniquely suited to improve balance and stability, improve posture, and increase lung capacity. Tai Chi and Qigong are built on two philosophical premises: First, that we are encouraging the healthy flow of energy, or Qi, through the body. Second that we are encouraging the balance of opposing forces, yin and yang, within the body. There are many different styles of Qigong and Tai Chi, so every instructor and every class will be different. Qigong exercises are often considered foundational to Tai Chi, as preparatory energy work, but they can also be done on their own as gentle energy exercise. Tai Chi is like a beautifully choreographed dance, with moves and patterns that you memorize, so it's easier to learn in a live class. We'll primarily focus this session on Qigong, to get you started with qi-based energy work. I encourage you to look for a Tai Chi class in your area. In many cities, you may even be able to find an outdoor class in a park, which is the best way practice.

Let's begin. We'll start in standing position, feet spread about hip-width apart, toes pointed forward, knees gently flexed. You can also practice this routine while seated, focusing on upper-body movement and your breath. We will offer insets of seated modifications throughout the practice, to support the adaptation of this exercise program into a seated exercise program.

Whether you are seated or standing, your arms are resting gently at your sides. Your shoulders should feel soft and relaxed. We'll begin with a focusing exercise, so close your eyes. Take your awareness within. Take a few deep breaths, breathing deep into your belly, letting your breath softly rise and fall through your body. Use your breath as an anchor, a focal point, to settle your awareness and let the rest of the world fall away.

We'll bring your hands onto your belly, centered over the belly button, one hand on top of the other, and focus on deep belly breathing, to help you center and calm and relax. Take an inhalation, and as you inhale let your stomach soften, let your lungs expand into the lower lobes of the lungs; let your stomach actually expand on your inhalation. As you exhale, contract your abdominal muscles—bringing the belly button back toward the spine—solar plexus lifting, air leaving your lungs. Inhale into the belly as it expands. Exhale, belly button back to the spine. Again, inhale. Exhale, belly button back to the spine, pushing the air out of the body, eyes are closed, awareness is within. Inhale. Exhale. Inhale. And exhale. A few more breaths. We tend to breathe shallowly—lifting our chest and shoulders as we inhale—but this constricts the lungs, tightens the chest, and leaves us feeling more anxious. Breathe like a child: Think about the soft, calming up and down of a baby's belly while sleeping. That's the kind of breath we are trying to re-learn, that same soft, fluid, natural breathing. Again inhale, use your hands as a physical reminder of the soft belly, exhale. Inhale, expansion of your lower lungs and stomach as you inhale completely. Your belly button back to the spine as you exhale completely. Inhale. Exhale. Inhale. Exhale. Inhale. Exhale.

Gently release your arms to your sides. Relax your legs, shake them out if you need to. The breathing can seem very simple but it's actually very powerful. It impacts how you feel, how you think; it can even affect your physical body. Deep belly breathing is good abdominal exercise. The Qigong instructor from El Paso, Texas that I mentioned in our introductory lecture had an incredibly strong core body, strong, muscular midsection, but he never did sit-ups. He just did deep abdominal breathing, consistently and deliberately, all day long every day. On your next inhale—as if there is a helium balloon attached to the palms of your hands, inhale your hands and arms up with your inhalation, pause at shoulder height, gently sink the arms back down as you exhale. Inhale. Exhale down. Through the nose, in and out as you breathe, remember to float your arms. Inhale, and exhale. You're moving as if through water. Inhale, exhale down. Your limbs are soft, flowing, moving gently. Inhale. Everything is round and circular, nothing sharp. Inhale, exhale. One more, inhale and exhale down. You want to challenge yourself a little bit more as you get strong, you can bend your knees gently into a gentle squat. Belly button back to the spine, strong core. Inhale up. Gently rotate your palms inward; let your elbows relax outward at shoulder height, as if you're holding a balloon. Pause here and exhale. Inhale, open up, open the arms, reach out, keep the elbows and fingers and shoulders soft. This is gentle expansion without strain. Exhale back together. Inhale open. Exhale float together. Inhale open. Exhale float together. Inhale open. Exhale together. Inhale open. Exhale together. Inhale open. Exhale together. Again, inhale open. Exhale together. One more time. Inhale, and exhale. And release your arms. If your knees are bent, straighten your legs, shake your legs out.

Let's gently warm up the joints. We'll start with the neck. Good, comfortable stance—your feet are wide apart and grounded. Arms are relaxed by your sides. As you inhale look up. Exhale, chin to chest. Gentle movement. Inhale up. Exhale, chin to chest. Inhale lift. Exhale chin to chest. Inhale lift. Exhale chin to chest. Inhale lift. Exhale tuck. Back up to the center. We'll inhale to the right, exhale to center. Inhale left, exhale center. Inhale right, exhale center. Inhale left, exhale center. Now bring your fingertips up to your shoulders; your arms are bent gently at the elbow. Begin making slow, small circles forward, as if you're swimming. Remember to breathe as you move. Gradually the movement becomes larger, shoulders moving more freely. Let your upper body move comfortably with your arms, let your hips flow along. Nice long stretch through the sides as the shoulders roll forward. Feel length in your torso. Then back to center and we'll slowly go the opposite direction, small circles at first, as if you're doing the backstroke now, gradually getting larger, getting wider with the circles, letting your torso and legs move with you. Remember to breathe, don't hold your breath, natural, fluid breathing. Then relax the arms.

Feet are a little bit wider apart, hands on your hips. Slowly circle the hips, small circle at first, gradually moving larger, as if you're hula-hooping. Be gentle with your knees; bend your knees as much as you need to to really take a nice circle pushing back, pushing forward, stretching the sides of the hips, stretching the back, the front of the body. And then pause and we'll start the other direction, again starting small, moving slowly to larger circles. If you're seated you're gently shifting your weight on the chair so that you can complete the rotation as well to continue to open up.

Then step your feet together. Bend slightly forward from the hips; hands are gently on your knees. If you're on the chair you'll need to come forward on the chair a little bit, again bending from the hips, hands on the knees. Rotate the knees gently, warming up the joints of the legs. Remember to breathe. Let it move comfortably through your ankles and your shins. Then gently move in the opposite direction; slow, comfortable circles. Then come back up to standing. Nice, solid wide stance. We're going to take ankle rolls. Hands are on your hips for balance. Lift one foot gently—roll the ankle, starting with small circles. You can move the circle bigger and bigger, moving your leg with the circle. If you're seated, you're moving one leg as well. Then rotate the opposite direction, starting small, moving bigger. Then relax, switch feet, start with the ankle, it gets larger, you can move the whole leg. Then going the other direction. And relax. Shake your legs out.

Nice wide stance. Arms stretch out wide in front of you; hands and fingers are soft and relaxed. Take wrist rolls at first, rolling the wrists in towards each other. Then roll away from each other. Wrist and ankle rolls are great to do throughout the day, keeping the joints open and fluid. Another simple thing that you can do at work while you're doing other things to keep movement throughout your day. And relax. Now we're going to take hand stretches. Spread the fingers wide. Curl them in. Inhale, stretch your hands. Exhale, curl them in. If you're seated, or if you're comfortable and want to challenge your balance, you can stand on one leg and do toes too. If you're seated you can do both feet at the same time. Inhale open, exhale curl. Inhale open, exhale curl. If you're standing and doing one leg at a time, switch feet. Inhale open, exhale curl. Again, these kinds of stretches are great to do throughout the day, maintaining hand function and flexibility if you work on a computer a lot. If you have arthritis or carpal tunnel, great way to keep some mobility in your joints. And release it down.

Let's do shoulder shrugs, give ourselves a massage. Inhale scrunch up, exhale release. Good to do this whenever you feel tension in your neck and shoulders. Inhale up, exhale down. Inhale scrunch up, exhale release. Inhale scrunch, exhale release. Inhale scrunch, exhale release. Inhale scrunch, exhale release.

Feet are nice and wide, comfortable stance—palms relaxed by your sides, hands open. As you inhale—arms float up to shoulder height—palms down. As you exhale—keep good posture and your back straight, belly button back towards your spine, bend your knees as much as you feel comfortable,

303

pressing down through the palms of your hands. Palms turn up—inhale—lift your energy upward—straighten your legs. Exhale down. If you're seated, focus on maintaining good posture, inhale up, and work the arms. Down, and up. Down, and up. Down, up. Down, up.

Remember we talked about the strength of the core, the bottom, the legs, down. It's so important for helping you maintain independence for standing. Down. For getting up out of a chair. Up. For walking. Down. Up. This is a great exercise to support that. Down, and up. You can practice throughout the day to strengthen your lower body and help you keep your lower-body strength. Let's do one more. Down and we're going to hold it here for several breaths. Feel strength in your legs, your core, and up. Relax the arms, shake out the legs.

Let's make rain. Again, a nice solid stance—feet are hip-width and pressed firmly into the ground. Arms float up to shoulder height, straight in front of you, fingers are soft, dangling down. If you're seated, you'll focus on the upper body. You're going to gently allow your whole body to become soft— and then slowly, gently you're going to shake. Shake your arms. Shake your legs. Shake through your torso. Allow your breath to be soft and natural. Imagine that all of the stress in your body is raining out of your fingertips, leaving your body softer and more relaxed. Continue to softly, gently shake all of the stress out of your body. Remember to keep breathing. Then stop shaking, release your hands to your sides. Come back up to a comfortable posture; shake the legs out.

This may not seem like much, but these kinds of simple, movement-based exercises are great for strengthening and toning the whole body. I did a drum circle workshop years ago, and the drum circle leader was an older woman who was very toned and in great shape—none of the flabby upper arm issues that often show up on women,= as we get older. Her main exercise was just drumming—but that standing, holding the drum between her legs, gently bouncing to the rhythm as she drummed—worked her muscles and toned her whole body. This connects back to motivation. It's important that our fitness be fun. It can be something as fun as drumming, but if your body is in it, it's exercise.

So don't worry that this feels gentle—that it feels different from other things you've done—that it feels silly while you shake. It's fun, it's silly, it's gentle, but it's doing your body good without any stress or pain.

Now, let's move the clouds. Good wide stance—toes pointed outward, gentle squat, arms at your sides. Your tailbone is tucked under; your belly button is pulled in toward your spine to engage your core. Place one hand on top of the other, and inhale your arms up through the midline, fingers pointing downward, to shoulder height. Rotate your hands in to face each other and exhale—arms out wide to the sides—push the energy out. As you inhale pause here and stretch out wide, opening your fingers to expand your chest. Exhale—hands circle down and in, back together in front of your groin. Inhale up, exhale open. Inhale stretch, exhale down. Inhale up, exhale open. Inhale stretch, exhale down. Inhale, exhale open. Inhale stretch, exhale down. Now straighten your legs, shake them out.

Now we're going to make a rainbow. A slightly wider stance. As you inhale, bring your arms up above your head, palms facing each other, elbows soft. As you exhale, shift your weight to your left leg, bending your left knee—let your right leg relax out to the side, and your arms gently stretch over the right leg. Inhale back to center, centering your weight. Arms up over the head, and then shift your weight to the right foot, bending the right knee, left leg relaxes out as you exhale over the left leg. Inhale up to center, exhale over the right leg. Inhale up to center, exhale over the left leg. Inhale up to center, exhale over the right leg. If you're seated, you're shifting your weight on your hip as you flow with your arm movements. You're still making the rainbow, moving your center of gravity. Inhale center, exhale stretch. Inhale center, exhale stretch. Inhale center, exhale stretch. Inhale back up. Relax your arms, shake them out, shake out your legs.

Now we're going to bounce the magic ball. Your feet are nice, wide, comfortable. Imagine that you have a very bouncy ball in your hands which is magic in that it can help you feel light and lifted. You're going to press down through your right hand while gently bending your knees to bounce the ball, and then with your right hand stretch up high over your head to your right side to catch the ball. Stretch so long your left foot lifts off the ground and you balance on your right foot. Bring your arm back down, foot back to the ground, ball in your left hand. Stretch high to catch it, right foot leaves the ground. Bounce, and stretch. Bounce, and stretch. As it becomes more comfortable, you can stretch farther with the fingertips, lengthen out more with the arms. Bounce, stretch. Bounce, stretch. If you're seated you're still stretching and lengthening, you can point the toe to the side. Bounce, and stretch. Bounce, and stretch. Couple more. Bounce and lengthen. Bounce and lengthen. Bounce and lengthen. Bounce and lengthen. Back to center; shake the arms out.

Now we're going to polish the golden table. Again, nice wide stance. Inhale your arms float up. Settle your arms and hands with your palms spread wide and open, and then bring them face down about waist height. We're going to step forward and out with the right foot, so you sweep your arms toward the right in a circle, as if you're polishing a table. Come back to center; step forward and out with your left foot, sweep your arms to the left. Back to center. To the right, you're polishing the table. Back to center, polishing the table in the other direction. Whenever your arms come back to your body, you're bringing your foot back to center. Sweeping left, and sweeping right. If you're seated, you're moving forward, stretching through the arms. If you're comfortable you can even shift your weight and lunge a little bit from the chair. Breath is expansive, gently flowing with your movement. Couple more, really lengthen and stretch and expand. And then come back to a centered, grounded posture and we'll do some kicks.

You're going to bring your arms to center in front of your groin, right arm crossed over the left. As you inhale, bring your arms up into a goalpost position, elbows bent straight out from the shoulders, fingers spread wide. Rotate your torso and your left foot so that you're facing the left with your weight on your right leg. Lift your left thigh up, balancing on the right foot. Kick through the left toe, and bring the foot down. Arms cross in front of your chest, return to center. Rotate right, open to goalpost, lift your right thigh, and kick. Then center, rotate, kick. Center, rotate, kick. If you're seated you can still be kicking, shifting the weight, working the legs. Center, rotate, lift and kick. Center, rotate, lift and kick. You're moving slowly. Deliberately. Lift and kick. Center, rotate, lift and kick. Center, rotate, lift and kick. Center, rotate, lift and kick. Back to center, relax down.

Step your feet together for a moment. Shake out the legs; shake out the arms. Now let's expand the golden ball. We're going to focus on our energy, learning how to actually feel the energy in the body. Stand in a solid stance, feet wide apart. Squat with your tailbone tucked in, your belly button pulled to the spine, to engage a strong lower body—we'll work to hold the squat throughout this exercise. If you're seated, focus on good posture, belly button to the spine, open chest, as we work with our energy. Shoulders are rolled down and back—your chest open. Bring your hands in front of you, fingers cupped slightly inward, as if you were holding a small ball in front of your waist. Focus your awareness on your hands—breathing in and out deliberately into the space between your hands. Take several deep breaths. Inhale, exhale. In and out through the nose, focusing on your hands. Inhale, exhale. Inhale, exhale.

Begin to be aware of the energy flowing from the fingers of one hand to the other. Inhale, exhale. It's as if there were invisible threads between your fingers. Inhale, exhale. Slowly as you inhale, open your arms and hands just a little. As you exhale bring them back to the ball you're holding in front of you. Breathing with the movement of your hands, but only move your hands as far apart as you can while maintaining the sense of connected energy, feeling the threads between your fingers. Feeling your wrists connected, your fingertips connected. We'll stay with this awhile—slowly inhaling and exhaling—creating openness in the chest, and connection in your body. Feel the expansion between your hands begin to grow; as you're able to keep your awareness of your energy, move your fingertips farther and farther away. At first you'll just keep your hands very small, but with practice, your fingertips will feel almost magnetic—pulling and pushing each other, and you'll begin to open wider and wider. Really try to feel the energy between your hands, keeping your focus on your fingertips, the pulsing of your blood, the warmth of your hands, feeling strings of connection grow longer as you slowly open farther and wider. Inhale, exhale. Inhale, exhale. Inhale, exhale. And then one more wide, expansive breath. And exhale, bring your hands back together, to the golden ball in front of you. Slowly straighten your legs and shake one leg out and then the other, still holding your ball.

And now we'll settle the chi; we'll bring it throughout your body, helping you to feel strong and well and energized in every part of you. All the energy in your hands, open your hands wide out to the side. As you inhale, sweep up and out, over your head. As you exhale, your fingers spread wide, pointing towards each other, palms facing down. Sweep in front of your body, helping that energy to settle in. Inhale, open and out. Exhale, the energy settles down in front of you. Inhale open, exhale bring that energy down through your body, bringing the chi throughout you. Inhale open. Exhale, settle the energy down. Inhale open. Exhale, bring that energy into your body. Inhale open. Exhale down. Inhale open. Exhale down. Inhale open. Exhale down. One more, inhale open wide. Exhale, bring all of that energy down into your body to feel strong and energized, and release your hands. Shake your legs. Settle your arms beside you.

Feel a sense of being strong and energized throughout your body, aware of your chi, aware of your energy. Feel a sense of awareness of how you moved your energy to promote blood flow through your body—to open your joints and improve balance, range of motion, and strength. We did gentle exercise, but it can have profound benefits for your health and well-being. Try this workout a couple of times per week to continue to build your balance, your strength, and the power of your own energy.

Bibliography

Books, DVDs, and CDs:
American College of Sports Medicine, ed. *ACSM's Complete Guide to Fitness and Health*. Champaign, IL: Human Kinetics, 2011.

————, ed. *ACSM's Exercise Management for Persons with Chronic Diseases and Disabilities*. 3rd ed. Champaign, IL: Human Kinetics, 2009.

Anding, Roberta. *Nutrition Made Clear*. Chantilly, VA: The Teaching Company, 2009.

Archer, Shirley, and Chuck Gonzales. *Fitness 9 to 5: Easy Exercises for the Working Week*. San Francisco, CA: Chronicle Books, 2006.

Austin, Denise. *Pilates for Every Body: Strengthen, Lengthen, and Tone—with This Complete 3-Week Body Makeover*. Emmaus, PA: Rodale, 2003.

Baechle, Thomas R., and Wayne Westcott. *Fitness Professional's Guide to Strength Training Older Adults*. 2nd ed. Champaign, IL: Human Kinetics, 2010.

Bandura, Albert. *Self-Efficacy: The Exercise of Control*. New York: Worth Publishers, 1997. Bandura's work is foundational to modern motivation theory.

Baumeister, Roy, and John Tierney. *Willpower: Rediscovering the Greatest Human Strength*. New York: Penguin Books, 2012.

Benson, Herbert. *The Relaxation Response*. New York: HarperTorch, 2000.

Bonura, Kimberlee Bethany. *Pelvic Yoga: An Integrated Program of Pelvic Floor Exercise to Overcome Incontinence and Support Overall Pelvic Floor Health*. Seattle, WA: CreateSpace, 2013. If you are working on pelvic floor strength to prevent incontinence, this book outlines the core components of pelvic floor exercises and provides detailed instructions and exercises for integrating them into your fitness program.

Brill, Patricia. *Functional Fitness for Older Adults*. Champaign, IL: Human Kinetics, 2004.

Buder, Sister Madonna. *The Grace to Race: The Wisdom and Inspiration of the 80-Year-Old World Champion Triathlete Known as the Iron Nun*. New York: Simon and Schuster, 2010.

Carrol, Cain, and W. D. Lori Kimata. *Partner Yoga: Making Contact for Physical, Emotional, and Spiritual Growth*. Emmaus, PA: Rodale, 2008. A physical approach to support connection.

Christakis, Nicholas A., and James H. Fowler. *Connected: The Surprising Power of Our Social Networks and How They Shape Our Lives—How Your Friends Affect Everything You Feel, Think, and Do*. New York: Back Bay Books, 2011.

Cohen, Kenneth S. *The Way of Qigong: The Art and Science of Chinese Energy Healing*. New York: Wellspring/Ballantine, 1999.

Cozolino, Louis. *The Healthy Aging Brain: Sustaining Attachment, Attaining Wisdom*. New York: W. W. Norton and Company, 2008.

Deci, Edward L., and Richard Flaste. *Why We Do What We Do*. New York: Penguin Books, 1996. Deci is the original researcher who developed the theory of self-determination.

Epstein, Lawrence, and Steven Mardon. *The Harvard Medical School Guide to a Good Night's Sleep*. New York: McGraw-Hill, 2006.

Gardner-Nix, Jackie, and Jon Kabat-Zinn. *The Mindfulness Solution to Pain: Step-by-Step Techniques for Chronic Pain Management*. Oakland, CA: New Harbinger Publications, 2009.

Hart, William. *The Art of Living: Vipassana Meditation, as Taught by S. N. Goenka.* New York: HarperOne, 2009.

Heller, H. Craig. *Secrets of Sleep Science: From Dreams to Disorders.* Chantilly, VA: The Teaching Company, 2013.

Iynegar, B. K. S. *Light on Pranayama: The Yogic Art of Breathing.* New York: The Crossroad Publishing Company, 1985.

Kabat-Zinn, Jon. *Mindfulness for Beginners: Reclaiming the Present Moment—and Your Life.* Louisville, CO: Sounds True, 2011. Mindfulness-based stress reduction is a research-proven approach to mindfulness.

Kasl, Charlotte. *If the Buddha Dated: A Handbook for Finding Love on a Spiritual Path.* New York: Penguin Books, 1999.

———. *If the Buddha Married: Creating Enduring Relationships on a Spiritual Path.* New York: Penguin Books, 2001.

Kneale, Angela. *Desk Pilates: Living Pilates Every Day.* Minneapolis, MN: Orthopedic Physical Therapy Products, 2008.

Kornfield, Jack. *The Inner Art of Meditation.* Louisville, CO: Sounds True, 1993. This audio CD is a favorite for learning the basics of meditation. Kornfield is an ordained Buddhist monk and a clinical psychologist; thus, he brings a unique combination of Eastern and Western skillsets to the teaching of insight meditation.

Langer, Ellen J. *Counterclockwise: Mindful Health and the Power of Possibility.* New York: Ballantine Books, 2009.

Levine, James A. *Move a Little, Lose a Lot: New N.E.A.T. Science Reveals How to Be Thinner, Happier, and Smarter.* New York: Crown Archetype, 2009. More about applying the principles of non-exercise activity thermogenesis to support health and wellness.

Maine, Margo. *The Body Myth: Adult Women and the Pressure to Be Perfect.* Hoboken, NJ: Wiley, 2005.

McGonigal, Kelly. *The Willpower Instinct: How Self-Control Works, Why It Matters, and How You Can Get More of It.* New York: Avery, 2011.

Muesse, Mark W. *Practicing Mindfulness: An Introduction to Meditation.* Chantilly, VA: The Teaching Company, 2011.

Paul, Marla. *The Friendship Crisis: Finding, Making and Keeping Friends When You're Not a Kid Anymore.* Emmaus, PA: Rodale Books, 2005.

Pink, Daniel H. *Drive: The Surprising Truth about What Motivates Us.* New York: Riverhead Books, 2009. An interesting and easy-to-read book on modern motivation theory.

Powers, Pauline, and Ron Thompson. *The Exercise Balance: What's Too Much, What's Too Little, and What's Just Right for You.* Carlsbad, CA: Gurze Books, 2007.

Prochaska, James O., John C. Norcross, and Carlo C. DiClemente. *Changing for Good: A Revolutionary Six-Stage Program for Overcoming Bad Habits and Moving Your Life Positively Forward.* New York: William Morrow Paperbacks, 2007. A great review of the transtheoretical model of change/stages-of-change theory, from the researchers who developed the model.

Richo, David. *How to Be an Adult in Relationships: The Five Keys to Mindful Loving.* Boston, MA: Shambhala, 2002.

Sapolsky, Robert M. *Why Zebras Don't Get Ulcers.* 3rd ed. New York: Holt Paperbacks, 2004.

———. *Stress and Your Body.* Chantilly, VA: The Teaching Company, 2010.

Schatz, Mary Pullig. *Back Care Basics: A Doctor's Gentle Yoga Program for Back and Neck Pain Relief.* Berkeley, CA: Rodmell Press, 1992.

Stein, Diane. *Essential Reiki: A Complete Guide to an Ancient Healing Art.* Berkeley, CA: Crossing Press, 1995.

Switzer, Kathrine. *Running and Walking for Women Over 40: The Road to Sanity and Vanity.* New York: St. Martin's Griffin, 1998.

Wayne, Peter M. *The Harvard Medical School Guide to Tai Chi: 12 Weeks to a Healthy Body, Strong Heart, and Sharp Mind.* Boston, MA: Shambhala, 2013.

Weil, Andrew. *Healthy Aging: A Lifelong Guide to Your Well-Being.* Norwell MA: Anchor Press, 2007.

Yee, Rodney. *Yoga: The Poetry of the Body.* New York: St. Martin's Griffin, 2002.

Zeer, Darrin, and Frank Montagna. *Office Spa: Stress Relief for the Working Week.* San Francisco, CA: Chronicle Books, 2002.

Web Resources:
American College of Sports Medicine. http://www.acsm.org/. Offers exercise information and updated news about exercise science.

American Tai Chi and Qigong Association. http://www.americantaichi.org/about.asp.

Chodzko-Zajko, Wojtek J., David N. Proctor, Maria A. Fiatarone Singh, Christopher T. Minson, Claudio R. Nigg, George J. Salem, and James S. Skinner. "American College of Sports Medicine Position Stand: Exercise and Physical Activity for Older Adults," *Medicine and Science in Sports and Exercise* (2009). Retrieved from http://journals.lww.com/acsm-msse/Fulltext/2009/07000/Exercise_and_Physical_Activity_for_Older_Adults.20.aspx. The full text of the ACSM position statement on exercise and older adults is available for free download.

International Association of Yoga Therapists (IAYT). http://www.iayt.org/. The IAYT publishes *The International Journal of Yoga Therapy*, a peer-reviewed scientific journal, focusing on yoga research studies.

Jack Kornfield. http://www.jackkornfield.com. Includes meditation practices and a blog from Kornfield.

National Center on Health, Physical Activity, and Disability (NCHPAD). http://www.ncpad.org. NCHPAD, a collaboration between the University of Alabama at Birmingham and several nonprofit organizations, provides a website specifically focused on physical activity for individuals with disabilities. The organization offers a 14-week plan; through a self-assessment on the website, participants receive free physical activity guidance targeted to their conditions. NCHPAD also offers articles about physical activity for a wide variety of chronic conditions and disabilities.

National Qigong Association. http://www.nqa.org.

National Senior Games. http://www.nsga.com. Learn more about the athletes in the National Senior Games and decide whether you want to join them.

Team Hoyt. http://www.teamhoyt.com. Get inspired by Rick and Dick Hoyt.

U.S. Department of Health and Human Services (USDHHS). http://www.health.gov/paguidelines/pdf/paguide.pdf. "2008 Physical Activity Guidelines for Americans." The full text of the USDHHS guidelines is available for free download.

Vipassana Meditation. http://www.dhamma.org/. Website of Vipassana Meditation as taught by the S. N. Goenka Organization. Offers resources and 10-day residential meditation courses.

Yoga Alliance. https://www.yogaalliance.org/. The Yoga Alliance is a national registry of yoga teachers. The site enables you to search for trained, qualified yoga instructors in your area.

Yoga Journal. http://www.yogajournal.com/. Website of the premier yoga publication. The site has substantial information available about yoga, including yoga poses, yoga practice guides, and yoga for specific conditions.

Notes

Notes

Notes

Notes

Notes

Notes